SUPER EASY VEGAN COOKBOOK

50 GORGEOUS BREAKFAST, SNACK, MEAL, AND DESSERT RECIPES FOR ALL OCCASIONS

VIRGINIA FARMVILLE

TABLE OF CONTENTS

---- BREAKFAST ----

---- LUNCH ----

---- DINNER ----

---- SNACKS ----

---- DESSERTS ----

Breakfast

RYE BREAD

Discover the beautiful flavors of homemade rye bread. You'll never buy it from shops again.

MAKES 8 SERVING/ TOTAL TIME 30 MINUTE

INGREDIENTS

1 cup (250ml) warm water

1 1/2 tablespoons treacle

2 teaspoons dried yeast

2 cups (320g) rye flour

1 cup (150g) plain flour

1 teaspoon salt

2 teaspoons finely grated orange rind

2 teaspoons fennel seeds

2 teaspoons caraway seeds

1/2 teaspoon ground cardamom

1/4 cup (60ml) extra-virgin olive oil

Caraway seeds, extra, to sprinkle

Fennel seeds, extra, to sprinkle

METHOD

STEP 1

Combine the rye flour, plain flour, salt, orange rind, fennel seeds, caraway seeds and cardamom in a large bowl and make a well in the center. Pour the yeast mixture and oil into the well and stir until mixture just comes together.

STEP 2

Use your fist to punch down the dough. Turn onto a lightly floured surface and knead for 2-3 minutes or until dough returns to original size.

STEP 3

Preheat oven to 220°C. Line an oven tray with baking paper. Shape the dough into a ball and place on the lined tray. Lightly brush with a little water. Sprinkle with extra caraway and fennel seeds. set aside in a warm, draught-free place for 30 minutes to 1 hour or until dough doubles in size.

STEP 4

Bake in preheated oven for 10 minutes. Remove from oven and set aside to cool.

NUTRITION VALUE

1192 KJ Energy, 8g fat,
7g protein, 43g carbs.

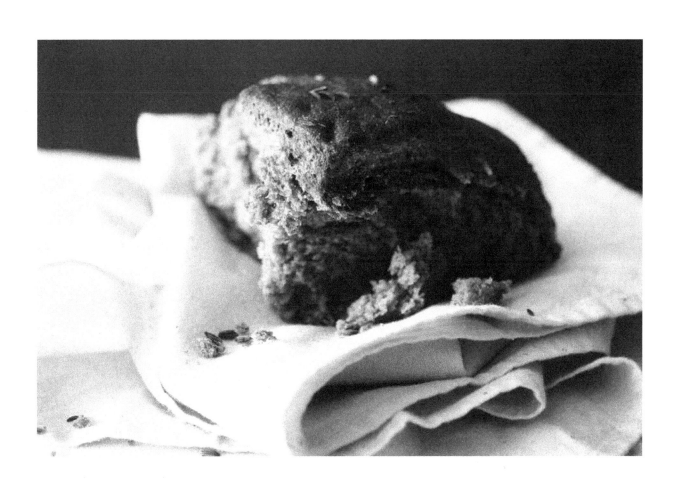

BASIC MICROWAVE JAM RECIPE

You won't believe how easy it is and this recipe is **vegan** friendly.

MAKES 8 SERVING/ TOTAL TIME 30 MINUTE

INGREDIENTS

1 lemon, halved

500g fruit (remove stone or stalk and chop fruit)

1 1/2 cups (335g) white sugar

METHOD

STEP 1

Juice the lemon. Place fruit, lemon juice and the rind halves in a large microwave safe bowl. Cook, uncovered, on High/100% power, stirring occasionally for 6 minutes.

STEP 2

Add the sugar and cook on High/100% power for 20 minutes or until the jam reaches setting point. (To do this, cool some jam on a chilled saucer and run your finger through it. If the jam wrinkles and stays separate it is ready to bottle.)

STEP 3

Discard lemon rind and spoon the hot jam into a clean jar. Invert for 2 minutes then turn upright to cool.

NUTRITION VALUE

1190 KJ Energy, 8.7g fat, 1.9g saturated fat, 13.6g fiber, 11.3g protein, 32.2g carbs.

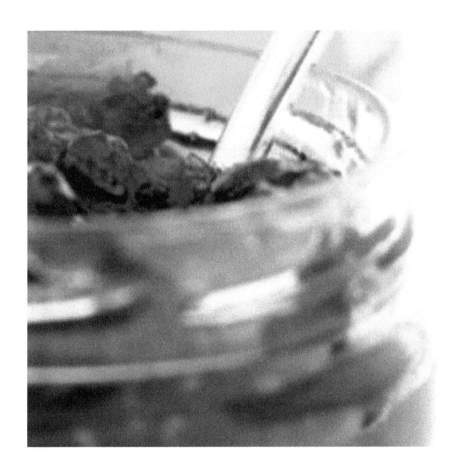

FRESH WATERMELON JUICE

This recipe is vegan friendly.

MAKES 6 SERVING/ TOTAL TIME 15 MINUTE

INGREDIENTS

1/2 (about 2.2kg) seedless watermelon, peeled, coarsely chopped

2 teaspoons finely grated ginger

2 tablespoons lemon juice

Mint leaves, to serve

Ice cubes, to serve

METHOD

STEP 1

Place watermelon, ginger and lemon juice in the jug of a blender and blend until smooth. Add sugar, if desired.

STEP 2

Strain through a fine sieve into a serving jug. Add mint and ice cubes and stir to combine. Serve immediately.

NUTRITION VALUE	491 KJ Energy, 1g fat, 2g protein, 24g carbs.

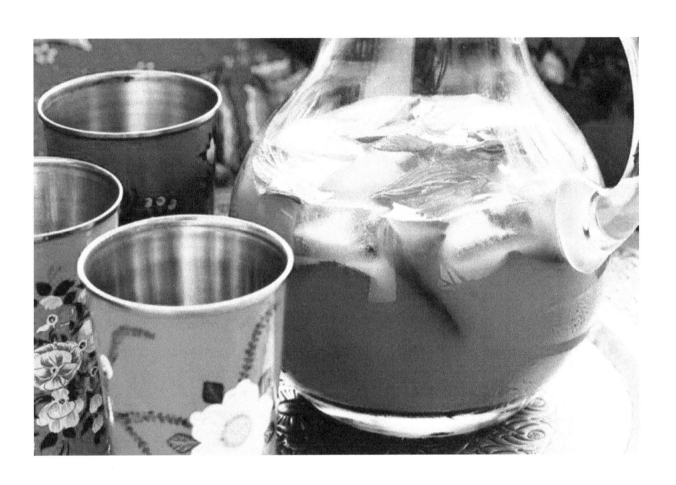

RED FRUIT SALAD WITH MINT SYRUP

Enjoy this refreshing dessert that doesn't take forever to prepare and goes down a treat with guests.

MAKES 4 SERVING/ TOTAL TIME 45 MINUTE

INGREDIENTS

1/3 cup caster sugar

10 large mint leaves

250g strawberries, hulled, halved

125g fresh raspberries

400g watermelon, rind removed, cut into 2.5cm cubes

METHOD

STEP 1

Place sugar and 1/2 cup warm water in a small saucepan over low heat. Cook, stirring, for 3 minutes or until sugar is dissolved. Add 8 mint leaves. Increase heat to medium. Simmer, without stirring, for 8 minutes or until mixture thickens. Remove mint leaves and discard. Set mixture aside to cool.

STEP 2

Finely shred remaining mint. Place strawberries, raspberries and watermelon in a large bowl. Toss to combine. Divide between bowls. Drizzle with sugar syrup. Sprinkle with shredded mint. Serve.

NUTRITION VALUE

549 KJ Energy,
3g fiber, 2g protein, 28g carbs.

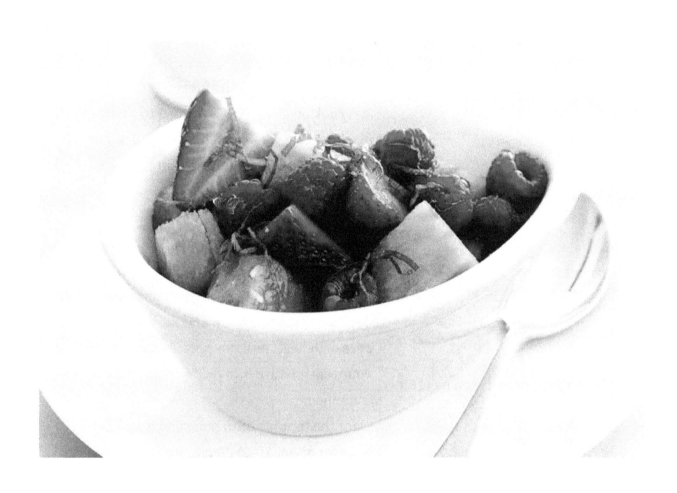

VEGAN APPLE AND BLACKBERRY CRUMBLE (FAT FREE)

This vegan apple and blackberry crumble tastes great and is a super healthy dessert or breakfast. We prefer to eat it cold with some plant milk.

MAKES 4 SERVING/ TOTAL TIME 35 MINUTE

INGREDIENTS

For the fruit layer:

2 peeled and diced apples*

2 cups fresh or frozen blackberries (300 g)

4 tbsp brown or coconut sugar**

1 tsp cinnamon powder

1 tbsp lemon juice

2 tbsp water

For the topping:

1 1/3 cup rolled or instant oats (160 g)

1 tsp ground cinnamon

3 tbsp agave or maple syrup

3 tbsp brown or coconut sugar

METHOD

STEP 1

Place all the ingredients for the fruit layer in a saucepan and cook over high heat. Bring it to a boil and then cook over medium-high heat for about 10 minutes or until the fruit is cooked. Pour the fruit layer into a baking dish and set aside.

STEP 2

Preheat the oven to 355ºF or 180ºC.

In the meanwhile, we're going to make the topping. Place the oats and the ground cinnamon in a mixing bowl and heat the syrup and the sugar in a saucepan over high heat until the sugar is melted. Stir frequently. Pour this mixture into the bowl and mix until well combined.

Place the topping onto the fruit layer.

Bake for about 10 to 20 minutes or until golden brown. And the crumble is ready to eat!

NUTRITION VALUE

164 Energy, 1.1g fat, 0.2g saturated fat, 5.3g fiber, 2g protein, 39.1g carbs.

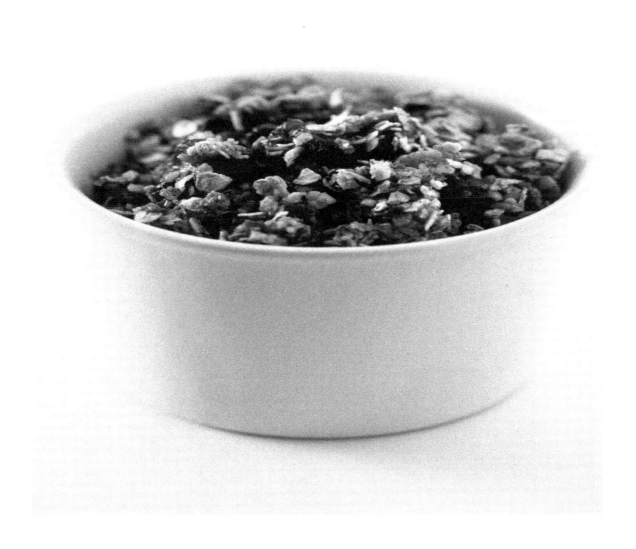

3-INGREDIENT VEGAN GF PANCAKES

These vegan pancakes are a great healthy breakfast, whether you like sweet or savory.

MAKES 6 SERVING/ TOTAL TIME 20 MINUTE

INGREDIENTS

1 banana

1 cup instant oats (100 g)

3/4 cup plant milk of your choice (185 ml), we used oat milk

METHOD

STEP 1

Grind the instant oats in a blender.

Add the rest of the ingredients and blend until smooth.

Place ¼ cup of the batter in a non-stick skillet (or a lightly greased skillet) and cook for about two minutes for each side.

Serve with your favorite toppings.

NUTRITION VALUE

98 Energy, 1.5g fat, 0.2g saturated fat, 2.5g fiber, 2.9g protein, 18.9g carbs.

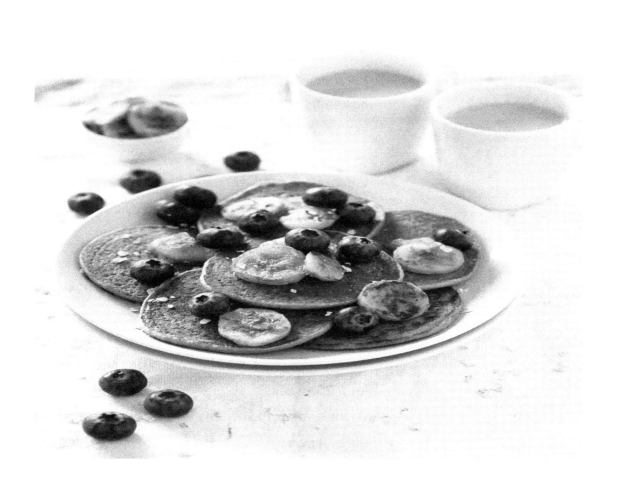

PEANUT BUTTER GRANOLA

Breakfast is the most important meal of the day, but you can eat healthy and also enjoy your breakfast. Try this peanut butter granola, it's delicious!

MAKES 8 SERVING/ TOTAL TIME 30 MINUTE

INGREDIENTS

For the granola:

2 cups oats (200g)

1/2 cup dried cranberries (75 g)

1 cup hazelnuts (150g)

2 tbsp water

1 tsp vanilla extract (optional)

2 tbsp coconut oil

1/3 cup maple syrup (100 g)

1/3 cup peanut butter (90 g)

For the jam:

1 cup blueberries (150 g)

2 tbsp water

The juice of a quarter of a lemon

6 tbsp coconut sugar

0.05 oz agar (1 g) (optional)

METHOD

STEP 1

Preheat the oven to 320 ºF or 160 ºC.

Place in a bowl the oats, dried cranberries and hazelnuts. Pour into a saucepan the water, vanilla extract, coconut oil, maple syrup and peanut butter, stir and cook over medium heat for 2 or 3 minutes

Combine dry and wet ingredients in the bowl and stir with a wooden spoon until all ingredients are totally mixed.

STEP 2

Place the granola on a baking sheet (with baking paper) and bake for 25 minutes.

Remove from the oven and allow the granola to cool completely. Place in a glass container and it should keep for a few weeks.

To make the jam you only have to place in a saucepan the blueberries, water, lemon juice and sugar and cook over medium heat for 30 minutes. You can add agar to thicken, but it's optional.

NUTRITION VALUE

346 Energy, 5.3g fat, 5.3g saturated fat, 5.5g fiber, 8.9g protein, 31.9g carbs.

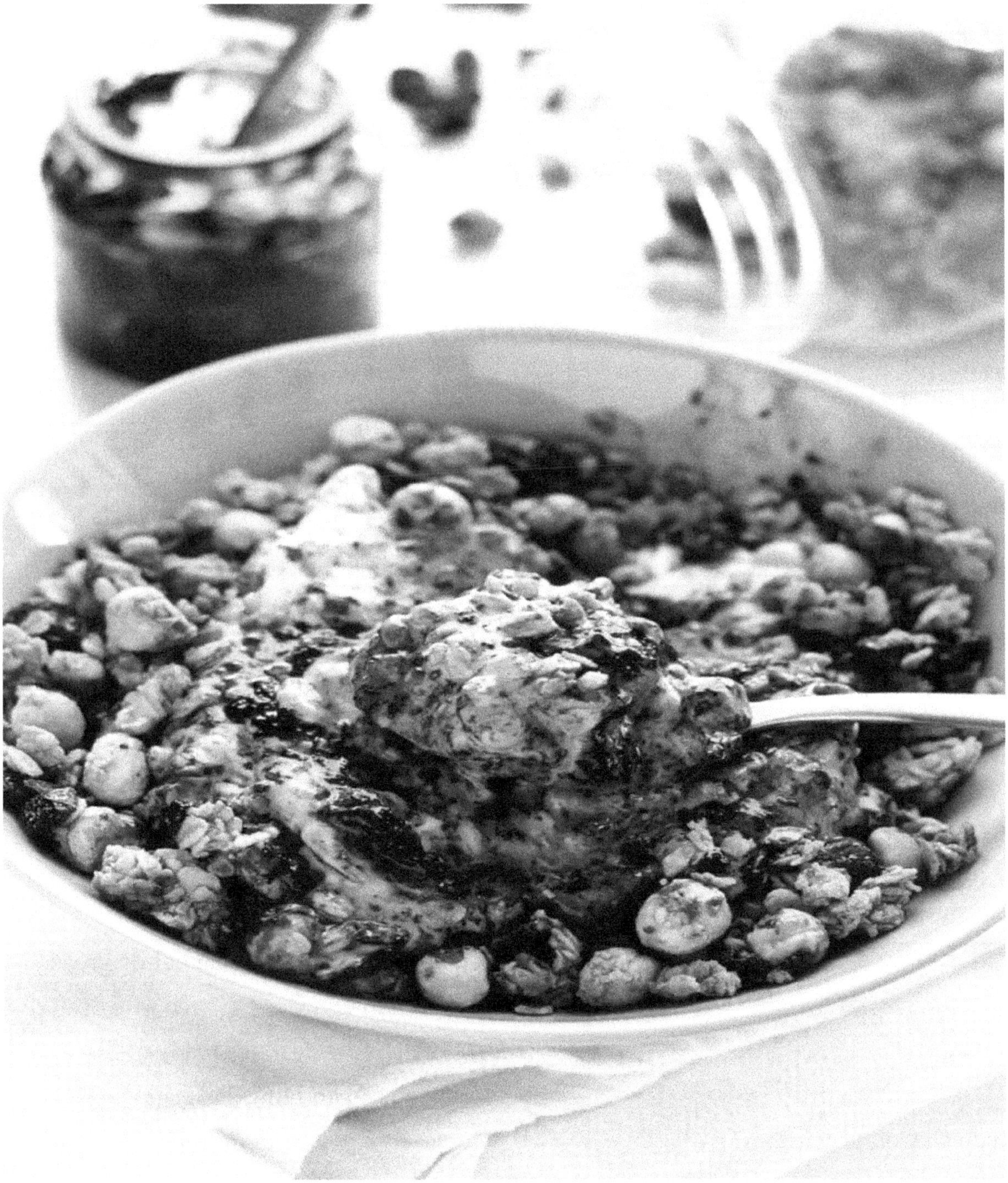

PUMPKIN CHOCOLATE CHIP PANCAKES

These pumpkin chocolate chip pancakes are vegan and gluten-free. They are the perfect pancakes and also lighter and healthier than traditional pancakes.

MAKES 9 SERVING/ TOTAL TIME 30 MINUTE

INGREDIENTS

1 cup chopped pumpkin or pumpkin puree (150g)

1 cup rice flour (150 grams)

1 cup oat flour (120 grams)

2 tsp baking powder

1 1/4 cups rice milk (300 milliliters)

2 tbsp maple syrup

1 tbsp coconut oil

1 tsp cinnamon

1/8 tsp ground ginger

1/8 tsp nutmeg

1 clove

1/2 cup chocolate chips (90 grams)

METHOD

STEP 1

Mix dry ingredients in a bowl (rice flour, oat flour, baking powder, cinnamon, ginger and nutmeg). You can make your own oat flour grinding oats in a food processor or a grinder.

Mix wet ingredients in another bowl (milk, maple syrup and oil).

STEP 2

Add the chopped pumpkin (or the pumpkin puree) and the wet ingredients in a blender and blend. Add the dry ingredients and blend again.

Pour the batter in a bowl, add the chocolate chips and stir with a spoon.

Place ¼ cup of batter in a hot pan lightly greased and cook for about two minutes for each side or until golden brown. You will know they are ready to flip when bubbles form on top and the edges appear dry.

NUTRITION VALUE

216 Energy, 6g fat, 3.7g saturated fat, 2.9g fiber, 4.7g protein, 36.7 carbs.

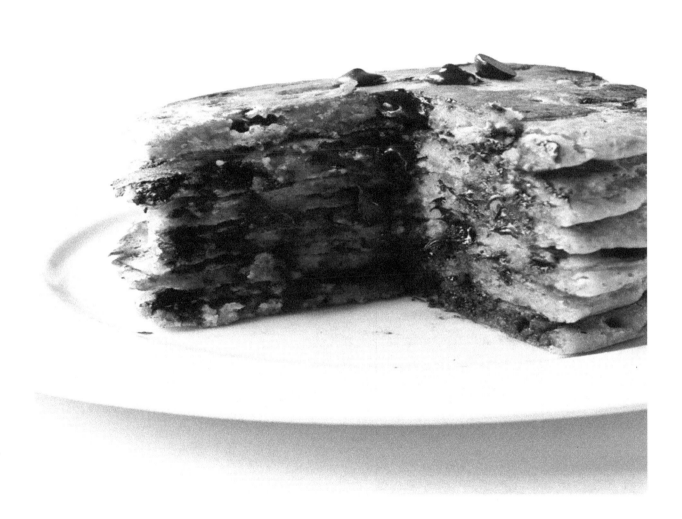

BANANA BLUEBERRY SMOOTHIE

This banana blueberry smoothie is the perfect breakfast smoothie, but you can also have it for lunch or dinner.

MAKES 1 SERVING/ TOTAL TIME 5 MINUTE

INGREDIENTS

1 banana

1 cup blueberries (150 g)

1 cup spinach (30 g)

1/4 cup oats (25 g)

1 cup plant milk of your choice or water*

METHOD

STEP 1

Place the banana, blueberries, spinach, oats and milk in a blender and blend until smooth.

Serve and your smoothie is ready to drink. Feel free to add any natural sweetener, like dates or coconut sugar.

NUTRITION VALUE

385 Energy, 6.1g fat, 0.9g saturated fat, 11.3g fiber, 8.4g protein, 79.1g carbs.

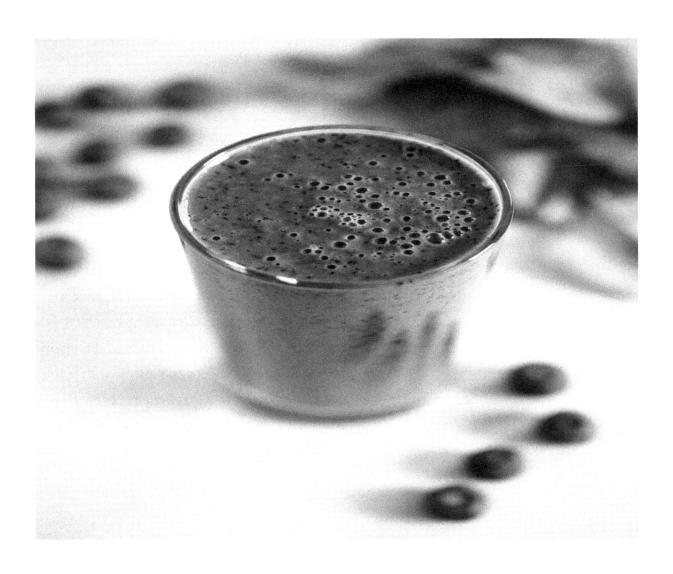

BREAKFAST POTATOES

Breakfast potatoes, made with 7 ingredients in just 30 minutes. They're so crispy on the outside, creamy on the inside, and super easy to make.

MAKES 2 SERVING/ TOTAL TIME 30 MINUTE

INGREDIENTS

1-pound potatoes (450 g), peeled if desired and diced

1–2 tbsp extra-virgin olive oil

2 tsp Italian seasoning or any other dried herb

1/2 tsp salt

1/2 tsp garlic powder

1/2 tsp paprika

1/8 tsp ground black pepper

METHOD

STEP 1

Preheat the oven to 400ºF or 200ºC.

Add all the ingredients to a large mixing bowl and mix until well combined (I prefer to use my hands).

Place the potatoes onto a lined baking sheet and bake for 20-30 minutes or until soft and golden brown

Serve immediately with sauces like vegan mayo, healthy ketchup, barbecue sauce, vegan aioli, and vegan sour cream. You could also eat them as part of a vegan brunch with fresh fruit, vegan butter, and homemade jelly toasts, tofu scramble, and natural orange juice or coffee. Another option is serving your breakfast potatoes with any vegan meat substitute like seitan or tempeh bacon.

NUTRITION VALUE	219 Energy, 7.3g fat, 1.1g saturated fat, 5.7g fiber, 4g protein, 36.2g carbs.

26

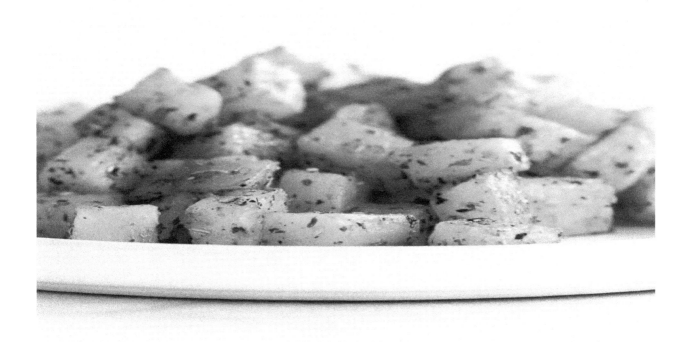

Lunch

SPICY ROASTED CAULIFLOWER RECIPE

Roasted cauliflower *is a fast and easy recipe that turns this unassuming and healthy vegetable into a star*

MAKES 4 SERVING/ TOTAL TIME 35 MINUTE

INGREDIENTS

teaspoon smoked paprika

¼ teaspoon turmeric

½ teaspoon garlic powder

½ teaspoon freshly ground black pepper

½ teaspoon fine sea salt

1 head cauliflower - cut into florets

3 tablespoons extra-virgin olive oil

Fresh parsley - chopped

METHOD

STEP 1

Adjust the oven rack to the middle position, and preheat oven to 425°F.

In a small bowl, add smoked paprika, turmeric, garlic powder salt and black pepper. Mix everything very well.

STEP 2

Place the cauliflower florets on an aluminum foil lined baking sheet. Pour olive oil on top of the cauliflower florets and toss until everything is evenly coated.

Sprinkle the spice mixture over the cauliflower, and mix well to combine.

Roast for about 25-30 minutes or until the cauliflower is tender and golden brown

Garnish with fresh parsley. Enjoy!

NUTRITION VALUE	111 Energy, 10.6g fat, 1.5g saturated fat, 1.9g fiber, 1.5g protein, 4.4g carbs.

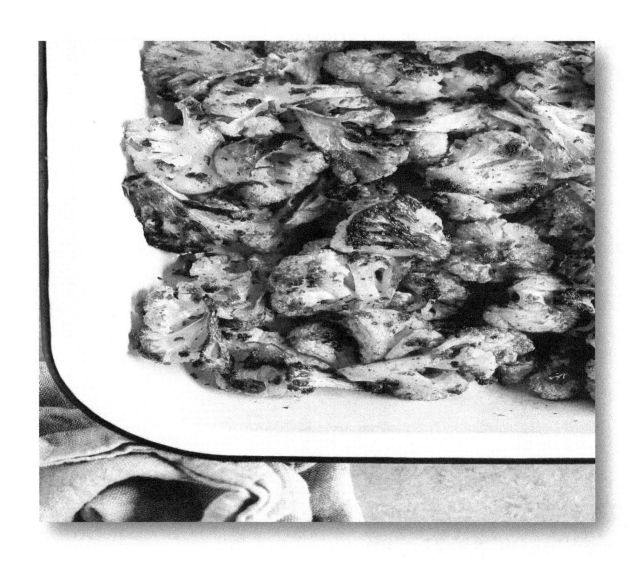

EASY ZUCCHINIS CAULIFLOWER RICE

Cauliflower rice *is a quick and easy way to replace starchy rice in any dish.*

MAKES 4 SERVING/ TOTAL TIME 10 MINUTE

INGREDIENTS

2 tbsp - olive oil

1 cup red onions - chopped

2 cups zucchinis - diced

1/2 tsp garlic powder

salt and black pepper to taste

5 cups cauliflower - cut into small florets

1 ½ tablespoon pesto

1 tbsp hemp seeds

Fresh parsley for garnishing - chopped

METHOD

STEP 1

Pulse the cauliflower florets in a food processor for about 25-30 seconds until it's a rice-like consistency. Set aside.

STEP 2

Add oil on pot or skillet over medium heat. Sauté onion for about 5 minutes. Then add zucchinis, garlic powder, salt and black pepper. Cook for about 4 minutes.

Add riced cauliflower and mix everything well. Cook until tender.

When it's time to serve, top with hemp seeds and fresh chopped parsley.

NUTRITION VALUE	180 Energy, 13g fat, 2g saturated fat, 4g fiber, 5g protein, 10g carbs.

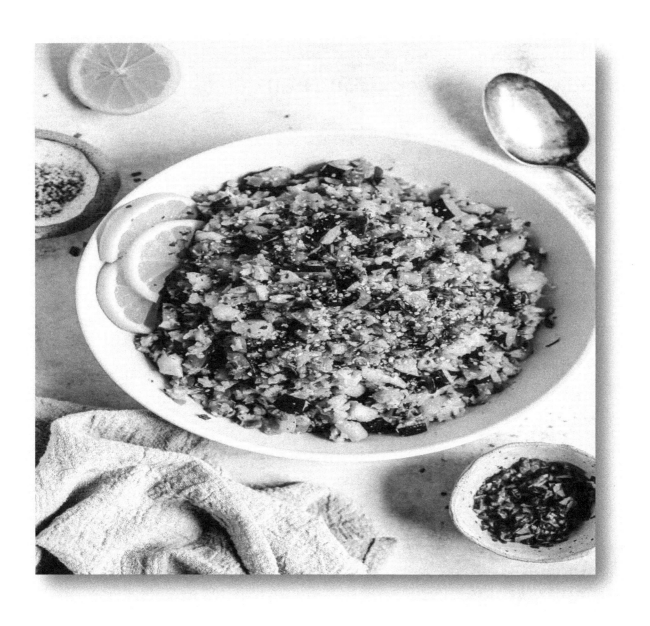

ROASTED BUTTERNUT SQUASH RECIPE

Roasted butternut squash is a delicious and healthy side dish recipe to make for lunch and dinner and serve with beef, chicken and fish.

MAKES 6 SERVING/ TOTAL TIME 20 MINUTE

INGREDIENTS

3 lb. butternut squash

2 tbsp olive oil

1/2 tsp salt

1/4 tsp black pepper

½ tsp paprika

Fresh parsley to taste

METHOD

STEP 1

Preheat oven to 425ºF. Line a baking sheet with parchment paper. Set aside.

Place butternut squash on a cutting board and using a vegetable peeler, peel your butternut squash.

Once it's peeled, cut your butternut squash in half and remove the seed.

STEP 2

Dice your butternut squash into bite-sized pieces roughly the same size so that they bake evenly.

Place butternut squash on the prepared baking sheet and drizzle on olive oil and season with salt, pepper and paprika.

Toss with your hands and then place in oven.

Roast for 15-20 minutes. Time will depend on the size of the butternut squash cubes.

Garnish with fresh parsley.

NUTRITION VALUE	143 Energy, 5g fat, 1g saturated fat, 5g fiber, 2g protein, 27g carbs.

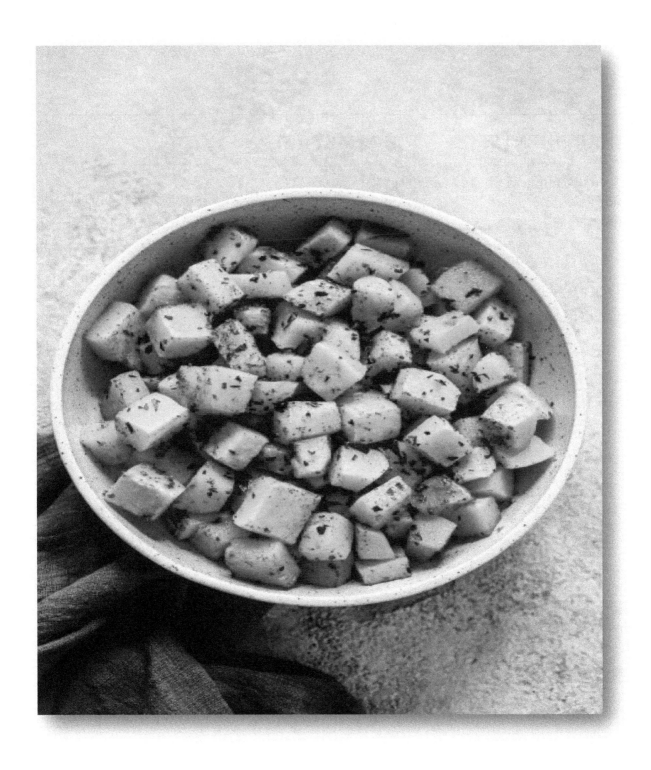

CAULIFLOWER "RICE" TABBOULEH SALAD RECIPE

Cauliflower "Rice" Tabbouleh Salad is an easy low-carb, gluten-free meal that can be prepared in advance making a great "on-the-go" lunch.

MAKES 4 SERVING/ TOTAL TIME 18 MINUTE

INGREDIENTS

1 small cauliflower head - cut off the florets

2 cups cucumber - chopped

2 cups cherry tomatoes - chopped

1 cup fresh parsley - chopped

¼ cup fresh mint - chopped

¼ cup olive oil

2 tablespoons fresh lemon juice

Salt and pepper to taste

METHOD

STEP 1

Pulse the cauliflower florets in a food processor for about 25-30 seconds until it's a rice-like consistency. Place the cauliflower in a microwave-safe bowl and microwave for 3-4 minutes. The time will depend on the power of the microwave.

Once cauliflower is cool enough to handle, transfer to a salad bowl.

STEP 2

Add cucumber, tomatoes, parsley and mint in the salad bowl. In a mason jar, pour the olive oil and freshly squeezed lemon juice. Add salt, pepper and whisk everything together. Continue to whisk while streaming in the olive oil. Taste to check the seasoning.

Pour the dressing over the salad, toss well and enjoy!

NUTRITION VALUE

188 Energy, 15g fat, 2g saturated fat, 5g fiber, 5g protein, 13g carbs.

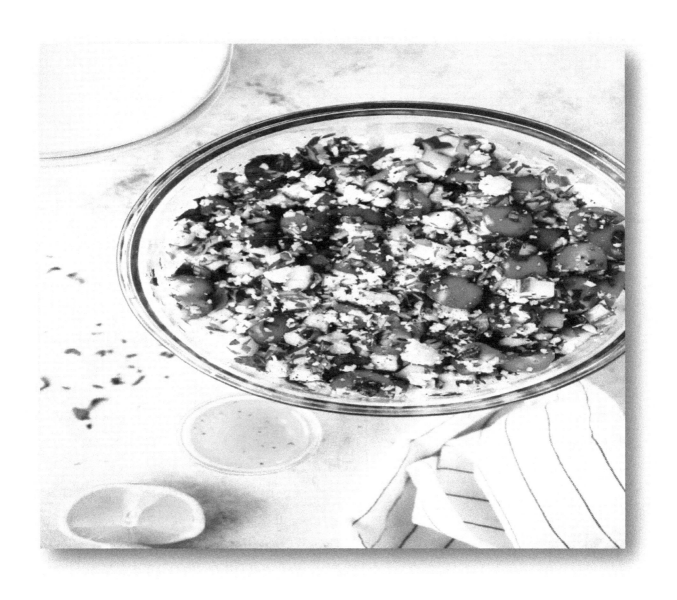

ROASTED RED BELL PEPPER PASTA

This Gluten-free Roasted Red Bell Pepper Pasta is also vegan, made with cashews, roasted red bell pepper, red onions, garlic and almond milk. And it's topped with crispy and super flavorful tofu.

MAKES 6 SERVING/ TOTAL TIME 20 MINUTE

INGREDIENTS

3 red bell peppers - roughly chopped

¼ cup red onions - chopped

1 clove garlic

2 tablespoons olive oil

½ package of Barilla Gluten Free Elbows Pasta

1/2 cup raw cashews

1/2 cup unsweetened almond milk

2 tablespoons nutritional yeast

Salt and black pepper to taste

Red pepper flakes to taste

12 oz. extra firm tofu

Chopped fresh parsley for garnishing

METHOD

STEP 1

Preheat the oven to 450 °F. On a baking sheet lined with parchment paper, mix the red bell peppers, onions, garlic and 1 tablespoon of olive oil and then spread evenly. Bake for 15-20 minutes.

Meanwhile, cook the Barilla Gluten Free Elbows Pasta according to the instructions on the package. Set aside.

In a blender or food processor, add the veggies from the oven, raw cashews, milk, nutritional yeast, salt, pepper and red pepper flakes. Blender everything until smooth If you think the texture is too thick you can add more milk according to your taste. Set aside.

STEP 2

Using a paper towel or a clean towel, press the excess moisture out of the tofu. Cut into small square pieces.

In a nonstick skillet, heat 1 tablespoon of olive oil.

Add the tofu and stir fry until golden brown. It's about 5-8 minutes. Set aside.

Place the pasta on a plate dish and top with the crispy tofu and fresh chopped parsley. Enjoy!

NUTRITION VALUE	309 Energy, 13.3g fat, 2.3g saturated fat, 4g fiber, 10.7g protein, 41.5g carbs.

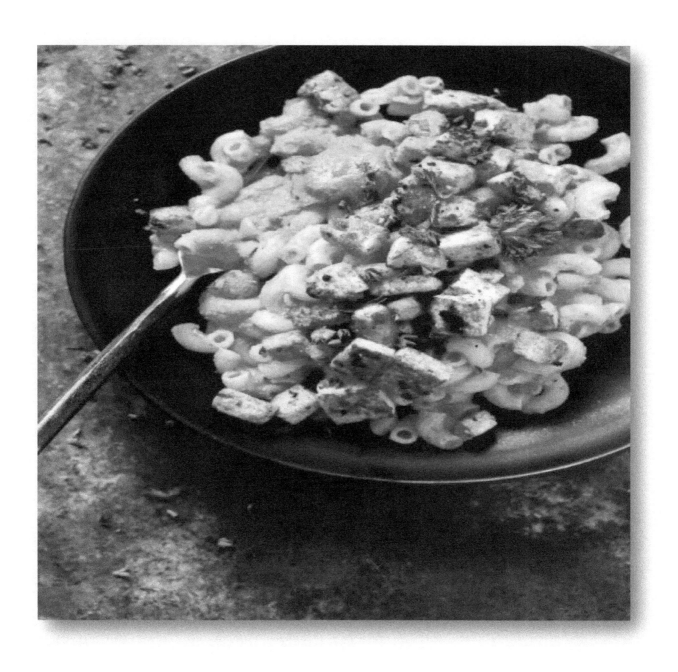

ROASTED BUTTERNUT SQUASH CAULIFLOWER SALAD

You'll love this Roasted Butternut Squash Cauliflower Salad for fall. It's tossed with an easy and very delicious vegan dressing.

MAKES 4 SERVING/ TOTAL TIME 30 MINUTE

INGREDIENTS

FOR THE SALAD

1 medium cauliflower head - cut into florets

1 small butternut squash - peeled and cut in cubes

1 tbsp olive oil

salt and black pepper

¼ cup red onion - chopped

1 tablespoon green onions - chopped

FOR DRESSING

1/2 cup veganaise or traditional mayonnaise

2 tablespoon yellow mustard

1 teaspoon garlic - minced

Salt and pepper

METHOD

STEP 1

First, steam the head of cauliflower. In a large pot add about 2 cups of water and place a steamer basket in the bottom. Bring the water to a boil. Add the cauliflower florets into the steamer basket.

Cover the pot and steam until the cauliflower florets are tender 6-8 minutes. Let the cauliflower cool down for 5 minutes.

STEP 2

Preheat oven to 400 degrees. On a baking sheet lined with parchment paper or silicone mat, place butternut squash and toss in olive oil and season with salt and black pepper. Mix well to combine.

Roast in the oven for 15-20 minutes

Place the steamed cauliflower, the roasted butternut squash and the red onions in a bowl.

In a small glass bowl, add all the ingredients for the dressing and whisk everything together to combine. Taste to check the seasoning and pour over the salad. Mix all the ingredients together until well combined and garnish it with green onions.

NUTRITION VALUE

287 Energy, 22g fat, 1.6g saturated fat, 5.5g fiber, 4g protein, 17.3g carbs.

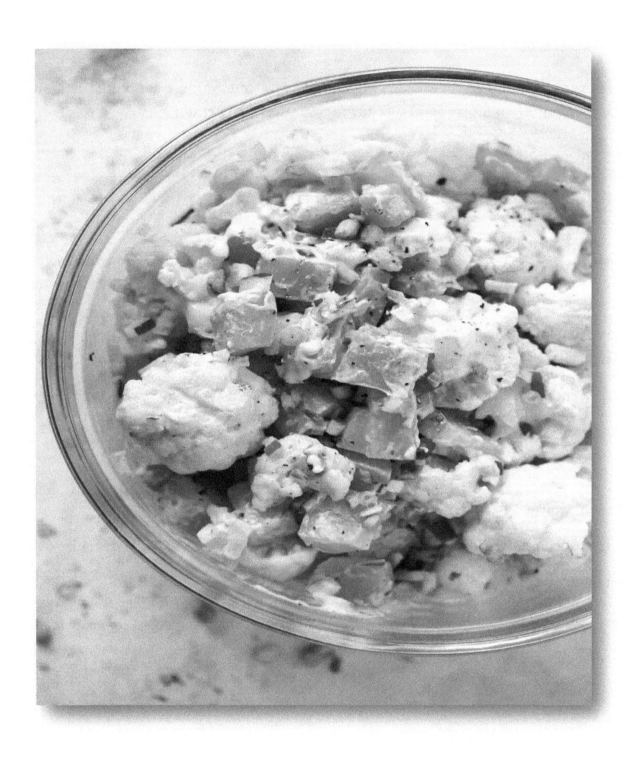

SUGAR SNAP PEA AND CARROT SOBA NOODLES

This recipe yields about six servings and the leftovers don't keep particularly well, so halve the ingredients if you're not serving a crowd.

MAKES 6 SERVING/ TOTAL TIME 30 MINUTE

INGREDIENTS

6 ounces spaghetti noodles of choice

2 cups frozen organic edamame

10 ounces sugar snap peas

6 medium-sized carrots, peeled

½ cup chopped fresh cilantro

¼ cup sesame seeds

Ginger-sesame sauce

¼ cup reduced-sodium tamari

2 tablespoons quality peanut oil

1 tablespoon toasted sesame oil

1 tablespoon honey or agave nectar

2 teaspoons freshly grated ginger

1 teaspoon chili garlic sauce

METHOD

STEP 1

Slice the carrots into long, thin strips with a julienne peeler, or slice them into ribbons with a vegetable peeler. To make the sauce: whisk together the ingredients in a small bowl until emulsified. Set aside. Pour the sesame seeds into a small pan. Toast for about 4 to 5 minutes over medium-low heat, shaking the pan frequently to prevent burning, until the seeds are turning golden and starting to make popping noises.

STEP 2

Once the pots of water are boiling: In one pot, cook the soba noodles just until al dente, according to package directions then drain and briefly rinse under cool water. Cook the frozen edamame in the other pot until warmed through and cook for an additional 20 seconds. Drain. Combine the soba noodles, edamame, snap peas and carrots in a large serving bowl. Pour in the dressing and toss with salad servers. Toss in the chopped cilantro and toasted sesame seeds. Serve.

NUTRITION VALUE	362 Energy, 12.7g fat, 1.6g saturated fat, 4.6g fiber, 17.2g protein, 53g carbs.

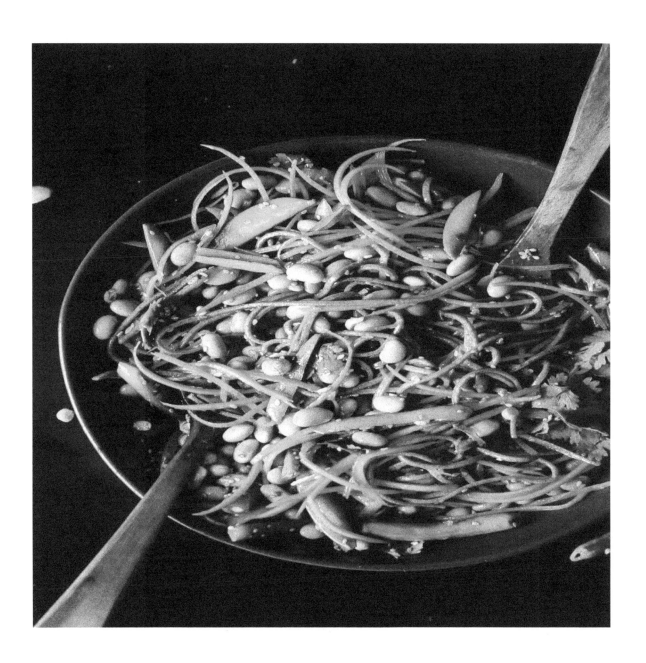

CREAMY (VEGAN!) BUTTERNUT SQUASH LINGUINE WITH FRIED SAGE

Serve with salad or roasted vegetables to further lighten up the meal. Recipe yields 4 large servings.

MAKES 4 SERVING/ TOTAL TIME 55 MINUTE

INGREDIENTS

2 tablespoons olive oil

1 tablespoon finely chopped fresh sage

2-pound butternut or kabocha squash, peeled, seeded, and cut into small ½-inch pieces (about 3 cups)

1 medium yellow onion, chopped

2 garlic cloves, pressed or chopped

⅛ teaspoon red pepper flakes (up to ¼ teaspoon for spicier pasta sauce)

Salt

Freshly ground black pepper

2 cups vegetable broth

12 ounces whole grain linguine

METHOD

STEP 1 Warm the oil in a large skillet over medium heat. Once the oil is shimmering, add the sage and toss to coat Add the squash, onion, garlic and red pepper flakes to the skillet. Season with salt and pepper. Cook, stirring occasionally, until the onion is translucent, about 8 to 10 minutes. Add the broth. Bring the mixture to a boil, then reduce the heat and simmer until the squash is soft and the liquid is reduced by half, about 15 to 20 minutes.

STEP 2

In the meantime, bring a large pot of salted water to a boil and cook the pasta until al dente according to package directions, stirring occasionally. Reserve 1 cup of the pasta cooking water before draining.

Cook over medium heat, tossing and adding more pasta cooking water as needed, until the sauce coats the pasta, about 2 minutes. Season with more salt and pepper if necessary.

Serve the pasta

NUTRITION VALUE	1190 KJ Energy, 8.7g fat, 1.9g saturated fat, 13.6g fiber, 11.3g protein, 32.2g carbs.

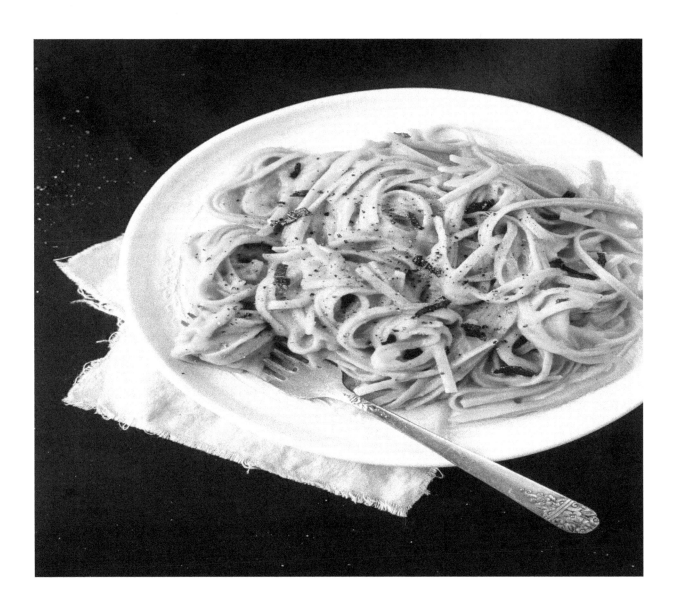

VEGAN SAUSAGE

Vegan sausage, a super convenient and tasty recipe It is 100% plant-based, delicious, and super flavorful, as well as perfect to eat for lunch or dinner!

MAKES 8 SERVING/ TOTAL TIME 1 HOUR 10 MINUTE

INGREDIENTS

1 tbsp extra-virgin olive oil, divided

2 cloves of garlic, sliced

½ onion, chopped

1 14-ounce can cannellini beans

1 tsp fennel seeds

1 tsp dried thyme

1 tsp ground cumin

1 tsp paprika

½ tsp salt

½ tsp ground black pepper

1 tbsp tomato paste

1 tbsp maple syrup

1 tbsp soy sauce or tamari

1 cup vital wheat gluten (120 g)

METHOD

STEP 1

Heat 1 tsp of extra-virgin olive oil in a skillet and cook the garlic and onion over medium-high heat until golden brown, stirring occasionally. Set aside.

Add all the remaining ingredients to a food processor bowl. Then add the cooked garlic and onion and pulse until well combined. Add the vital wheat gluten and pulse again until well combined and it comes together in a ball. It's okay if it's not a perfect ball.

STEP 2

Roll and press the dough into a sausage shape. Roll tightly each sausage in aluminum foil. Twist the ends so that each sausage is completely covered in foil.

Add the vegan sausages into the steaming basket and steam for 40 minutes, flipping them after 20 minutes. Remove from the stove and let them cool for about 5 minutes, then unwrap. Heat the remaining extra-virgin olive oil in a large skillet and then cook the sausages over medium-high heat for about 1 to 2 minutes on each side, You can serve your vegan sausages with BBQ sauce, mustard, vegan mashed potatoes.

NUTRITION VALUE

215 Energy, 2.1g fat, 0.3g saturated fat, 11g fiber, 19.6g protein, 32.2g carbs.

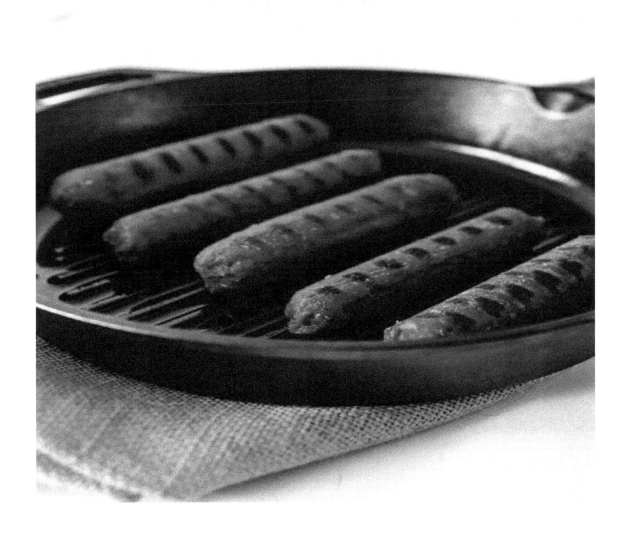

VEGAN POT PIE

Vegan pot pie, one of my favorite comfort recipes ever. It is super warm, cozy, and flavorful, as well as perfect to enjoy during the wintertime.

MAKES 8 SERVING/ TOTAL TIME 1 HOUR

INGREDIENTS

2 batches of vegan pie crust,

2 tbsp vegan butter

3 cloves of garlic, sliced

1 medium onion, chopped

1 celery stick, chopped

2 medium carrots, chopped

12 oz store-bought

⅓ cup all-purpose flour (40 g)

2 cups vegan chicken stock (480 ml),

½ cup unsweetened plant milk

½ cup frozen peas (65 g)

½ tsp salt

¼ tsp ground black pepper

2 tsp dried thyme

2 tbsp fresh parsley, finely chopped

METHOD
STEP 1
Preheat the oven to 400ºF or 200ºC.

Heat the vegan butter (or oil) in a large pot and cook the veggies (garlic, onion, celery, and carrots) over medium-high heat for about 10 minutes or until soft, stirring occasionally. Add the vegan chicken Add the Then add the vegetable stock and the plant milk and stir. After that, incorporate all the remaining ingredients, stir again and cook until it thickens, stirring occasionally.

STEP 2
Pour the filling into the pie crust-lined pan. I use a 9-inch or 23 cm round pie pan.

Roll the second vegan pie crust into a round and place over the pie filling. Fold the excess dough behind the bottom crust then crimp the pie crusts together to seal. Bake for 35 to 45 minutes Remove from the oven and let it rest for 15 minutes to cool slightly before slicing. and serve immediately with breakfast potatoes, roasted red peppers, or your favorite side dish.

NUTRITION VALUE

197 Energy, 8.4g fat, 2g saturated fat, 3g fiber, 9.6g protein, 32.2g carbs.

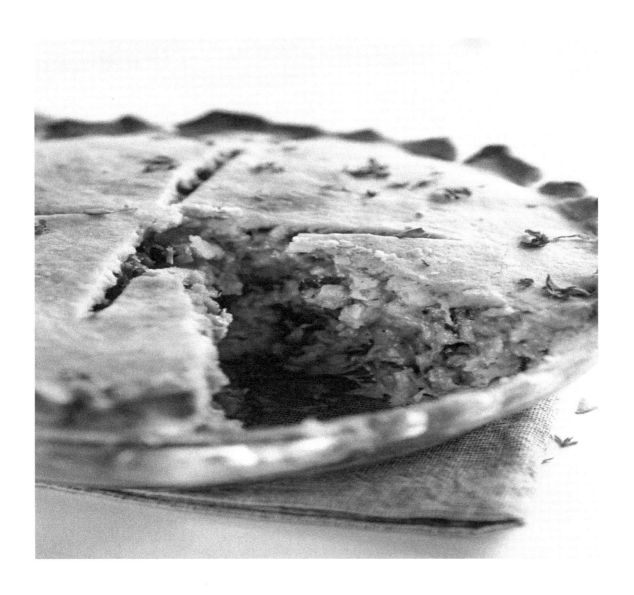

Dinner

SPICY CARROT SOUP

The perfect balance between spicy and sweet, this **Spicy Carrot Soup** *will warm you up on those chilly night.*

MAKES 4 SERVING/ TOTAL TIME 25 MINUTE

INGREDIENTS

1 tbsp olive oil
1 yellow onion
1-pound carrots - peeled and chopped
1/2 tsp salt
1/2 tsp freshly ground pepper
1/2 tsp curry
½ tsp coriander
¼ tsp cayenne pepper
1 tbsp garlic powder
4 cups vegetable broth - If you think it's too thick, you can add more.
Fresh parsley and peanuts for garnishing

METHOD

STEP 1

In a large soup pot over high heat, add olive oil. When the pan and the oil are hot, turn the heat down to medium and add the onions. Cook until onions are translucent.

STEP 2

Then, add carrots and all the spices (salt, pepper, curry, coriander, cayenne pepper and garlic powder.)

Stir all together to combine and add vegetable broth.

Bring it to a boil, cook with lid partially on, until carrots are tender. It is about 20 minutes.

Using an immersion hand blender or a counter-top blender puree the carrots. Taste and add any extra seasonings, if necessary.

Serve topped with fresh parsley and peanuts.

NUTRITION VALUE	117 KJ Energy, 4g fat, 1g saturated fat, 5g fiber, 11.3g protein, 32.2g carbs.

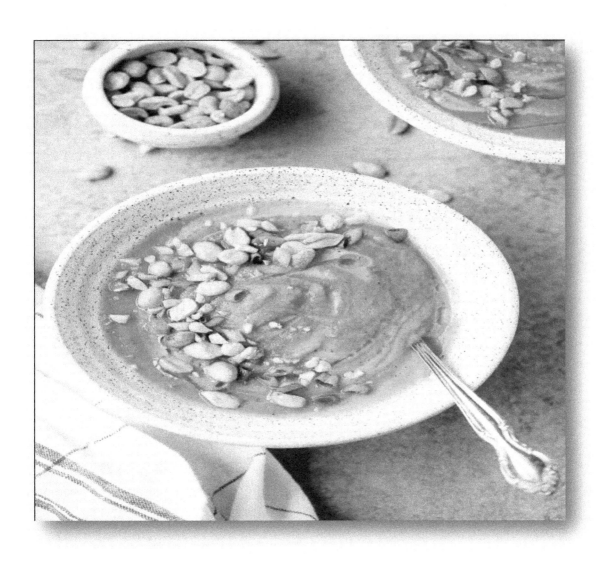

BALSAMIC ROASTED VEGETABLES RECIPE

Balsamic roasted vegetables make an easy and amazingly flavorful side dish.

MAKES 6 SERVING/ TOTAL TIME 40 MINUTE

INGREDIENTS

FOR THE ROASTED VEGETABLES

2 cups butternut squash - diced

2 cups radishes - cut them into quarters

1 cup parsnip - sliced

1 red bell pepper - cut into thick 1-inch pieces

1 cup zucchinis - chopped

1 red onion - cut into thick 1-inch pieces

fresh parsley - to garnish

FOR THE DRESSING

1/4 cup olive oil

2 tablespoons balsamic vinegar

1 tsp. dried basil

Salt and black pepper to taste

1 tsp. dried Italian seasoning

METHOD

STEP 1

FOR THE DRESSING

Combine all the ingredients for the dressing in a small mason jar. Close with the lid and shake well. Let sit while cutting vegetables.

STEP 2

FOR THE ROASTED VEGETABLES

Preheat oven to 425 degrees F. Line a large baking sheet with parchment paper.

Place butternut squash, radishes and Brussels sprouts on the prepared baking sheet. Spread into an even layer.

Shake the dressing and drizzle half of it over the butternut squash, radishes and parsnip. Toss to coat and roast for about 15-20 minutes.

Remove the baking sheet from the oven and add in bell pepper, zucchinis and onions. Return to oven and roast for more 15-20 minutes.

Before serving, top it with fresh parsley.

NUTRITION VALUE

176 Energy, 9g fat, 1g saturated fat, 4g fiber, 2g protein, 23g carbs.

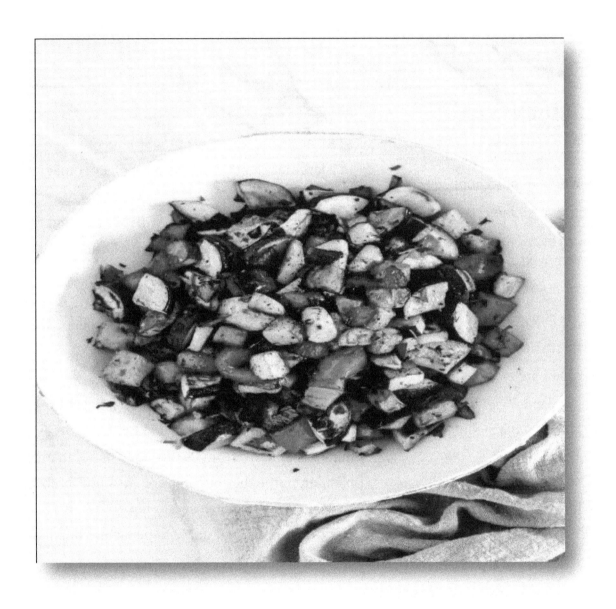

20-MINUTES BUTTERNUT SQUASH SOUP

20-minutes Butternut Squash Soup is a simple, easy and delicious side dish for a holiday dinner party or a quick healthy lunch to enjoy during fall cold-weather.

MAKES 4 SERVING/ TOTAL TIME 25 MINUTE

INGREDIENTS

1 1/2 tablespoons olive oil

1 cup white onion - chopped

3 garlic cloves - minced

2 pounds butternut squash peeled - seeds removed and cubed

1 teaspoon sea salt

1/4 teaspoon ground black pepper

¼ teaspoon turmeric

½ teaspoon paprika

1 teaspoon onion powder

1 1/2 cups vegetable broth - use less if you prefer a thicker soup

1 1/2 cups almond milk

Pistachios and fresh parsley - chopped

METHOD

STEP 1

In a large stock pot, heat the olive oil over medium high heat.

Add in the onion, stir to coat with olive oil and cook for about 2-4 minutes. Then, add in garlic and cook until the garlic becomes fragrant.

Add in the butternut squash, salt, pepper, turmeric, paprika and onion powder. Sauté for about 5-7 minutes. Stir occasionally.

STEP 2

Add in vegetable broth and almond milk, stir to combine. Bring to a boil and then to a simmer for another 10 minutes. Remove from the heat and using an immersion blender, puree the soup ingredients until combined and smooth. Taste to adjust seasoning.

Serve into bowls and top with pistachios and parsley.

NUTRITION VALUE	195 Energy, 6g fat, 1g saturated fat, 5g fiber, 3g protein, 6g carbs.

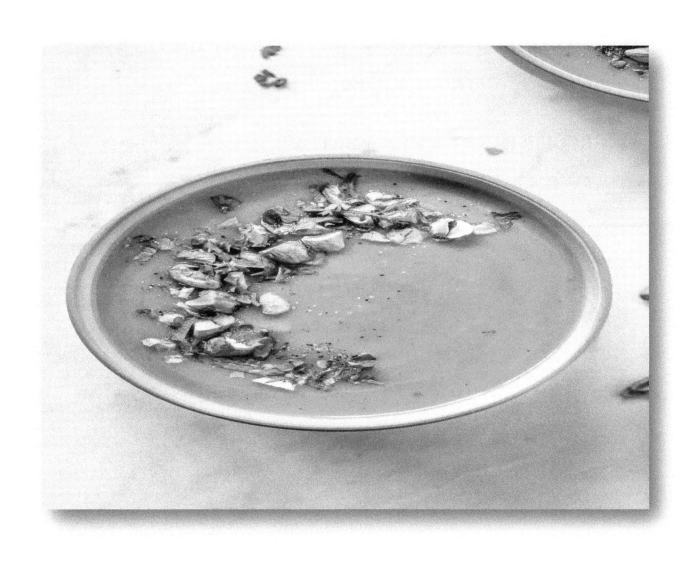

GOLDEN CAULIFLOWER RICE RECIPE

Golden Cauliflower Rice is a light version of traditional rice recipe and it's loaded with nutrients, vitamins and antioxidant. Perfect healthy side dish!

MAKES 4 SERVING/ TOTAL TIME 20 MINUTE

INGREDIENTS

1 head medium cauliflower rice

2 tbsp extra-virgin olive oil or coconut oil

½ cup small white onion - chopped

½ cup red bell pepper - chopped

1 garlic clove - minced

1-2 tbsp turmeric powder

Salt and ground black pepper to taste

Fresh chives for garnish - chopped

METHOD

STEP 1

Pulse the cauliflower florets in a food processor for about 25-30 seconds until it's a rice-like consistency. Set aside.

STEP 2

Add oil on skillet over medium heat. Sauté onion, red bell pepper and garlic for about 4 minutes

Add riced cauliflower and add turmeric. Mix everything well.

Cook until tender and season with salt and pepper to taste.

When it's time to serve, top with chives.

NUTRITION VALUE

131 Energy, 8g fat, 1g saturated fat, 6g fiber, 4g protein, 10g carbs.

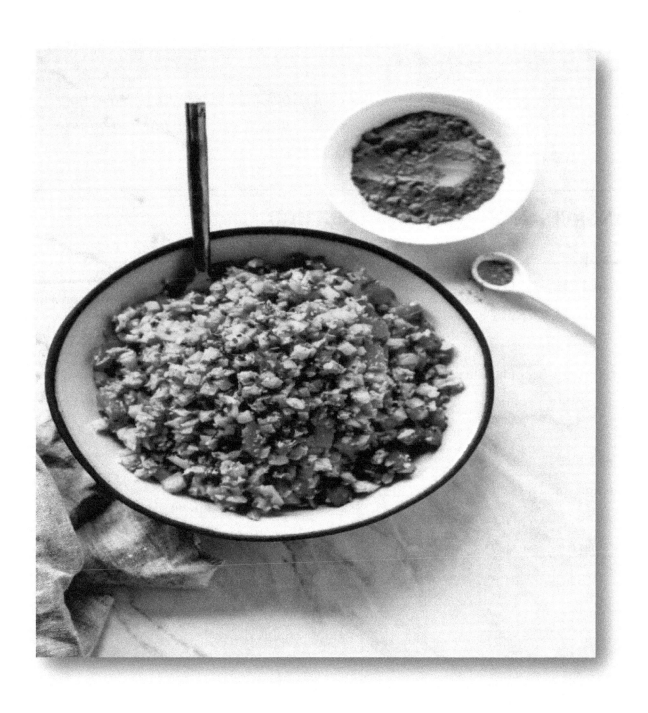

MUSHROOM CAULIFLOWER RICE SKILLET RECIPE

This Mushroom Cauliflower Rice Skillet is a delicious low-carb, paleo, whole30 and vegan/vegetarian main dish for dinner. And, it's done in only 20 minutes.

MAKES 4 SERVING/ TOTAL TIME 20 MINUTE

INGREDIENTS

2 tbsp extra-virgin olive oil

1 stick celery - sliced

½ cup onion - chopped

1 big garlic clove - minced

3 cups mushrooms - sliced

14 oz. 400g cauliflower rice

1/3 cup organic vegetable broth

Soy sauce to taste

2 cups spinach

Salt and black pepper to taste

1 tbsp fresh parsley - chopped

METHOD

STEP 1

Pulse the cauliflower florets in a food processor for about 25-30 seconds until it's a rice-like consistency. Set aside.

In a large skillet add olive oil over medium heat.

Add onions and celery and cook until tender about 5 minutes. Add garlic and cook for 30 seconds.

STEP 2

Add mushroom and sauté until it's cooked through.

Add the cauliflower rice, the vegetable broth, and soy sauce. Allow the cauliflower rice to absorb the vegetable broth. Cook until it is soft, but not mushy.

Add spinach and cook for 2 minutes. Season with salt and pepper to taste

Garnish with chopped fresh parsley before serving.

Enjoy!

NUTRITION VALUE

125 Energy, 7.3g fat, 1g saturated fat, 4.2g fiber, 4.6g protein, 9.8g carbs.

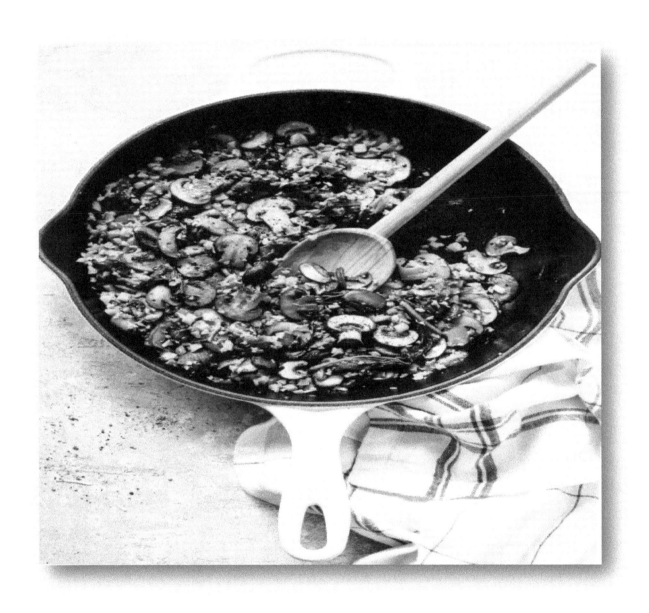

SIMPLE KALE SALAD WITH AVOCADO DRESSING

Simple Kale Salad with Avocado Dressing, which is so delicious, and it's done in 5 minutes by pulsing the dressing ingredients in a food processor.

MAKES 6 SERVING/ TOTAL TIME 15 MINUTE

INGREDIENTS

FOR THE SALAD

3 cups kale - ribs removed and leaves chopped

3 cups red cabbage - chopped

½ cup red onion - chopped

½ cup red bell pepper - chopped

FOR THE DRESSING

1 avocado

1 cup chopped parsley

2 cloves garlic

1 tbsp lemon juice

1/2 cup water

2/3 cup olive oil

1/2 cup pine nuts

Salt and black pepper to taste

METHOD

STEP 1

In a large salad bowl, add kale, red cabbage, red onions and bell pepper. Set aside.

In a food processor, pulse all ingredients until smooth. Add less water if you prefer your dressing creamer. The amount of water will depend on what consistency you want.

Taste to check the seasoning and pour over the salad. Mix everything very well. Enjoy!

NUTRITION VALUE	269 Energy, 24g fat, 3g saturated fat, 5g fiber, 4g protein, 13g carbs.

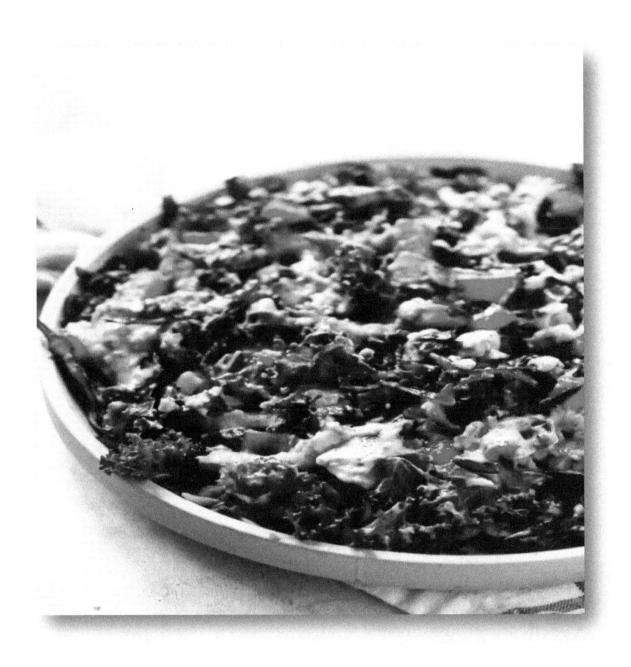

CHOPPED RED CABBAGE KALE SALAD

Easy, quick and delicious Chopped Red Cabbage Kale Salad to keep you healthy during the cold weather.

MAKES 4 SERVING/ TOTAL TIME 10 MINUTE

INGREDIENTS

FOR THE SALAD

3 cups kale - ribs removed and leaves chopped

3 cups red cabbage - chopped

1 small red apple - sliced

¼ cup sliced almond

FOR THE DRESSING

3 tbsp olive oil

1 tbsp lemon juice

1 tbsp balsamic

1 tsp Dijon mustard

Salt and pepper

METHOD

STEP 1

In a large salad bowl, add kale, red cabbage, red apple and sliced almond.

In a mason jar, pour the olive oil, lemon juice, balsamic, Dijon mustard, salt and pepper. Whisk everything together. Continue to whisk while streaming in the olive oil*.

Taste to check the seasoning and pour over the salad. Enjoy!

NUTRITION VALUE

179 Energy, 14g fat, 2g saturated fat, 4g fiber, 3g protein, 13g carbs.

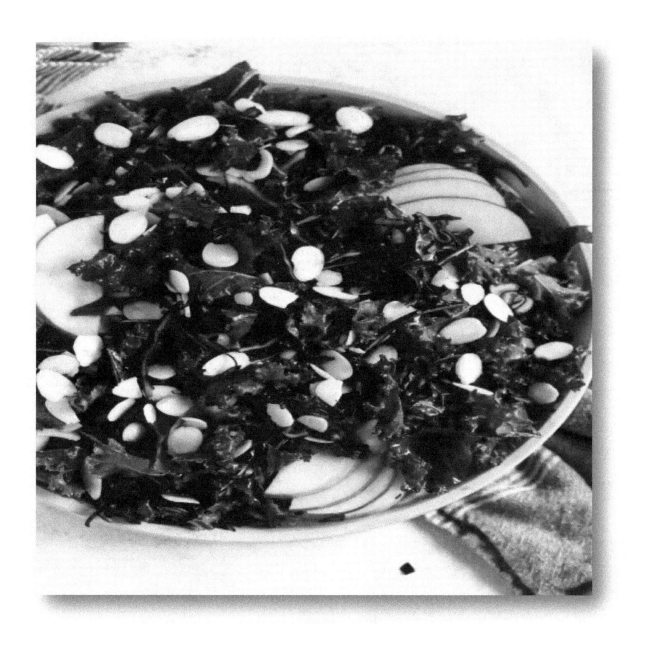

AUTUMN BEET ORANGE SALAD RECIPE

This Autumn Beet Orange Salad is flavorful, healthy, and effortless and it's tossed with a tangy orange mustard vinaigrette.

MAKES 4 SERVING/ TOTAL TIME 17 MINUTE

INGREDIENTS

FOR THE SALAD:

2 big red beets - peeled and cut in cubes

1 medium orange - peeled and cut in cubes

1/2 small red onion - sliced

5 cups green leaves - arugula, spinach and so on

1/4 cup chopped pistachios

FOR THE VINAIGRETTE:

3 tbsp fresh orange juice

1 tbsp lemon juice

3 tbsp olive oil

1 tbsp Dijon mustard

Salt and black pepper to taste

METHOD

STEP 1

In a small pot bring water to a boil and add the beets. Cook for about 5-8 minutes or until the beets are tender. Set aside.

STEP 2

In a large salad bowl, add all the ingredients for the salad and the cooked beets.

In a mason jar, pour the orange juice, lemon juice, olive oil and Dijon mustard. Add salt and pepper and whisk everything together. Continue to whisk while streaming in the olive oil. Taste to check the seasoning.

Pour the dressing over the salad and toss well. Enjoy!

NUTRITION VALUE

146 KJ Energy, 9g fat, 1g saturated fat, 4g fiber, 4g protein, 15g carbs.

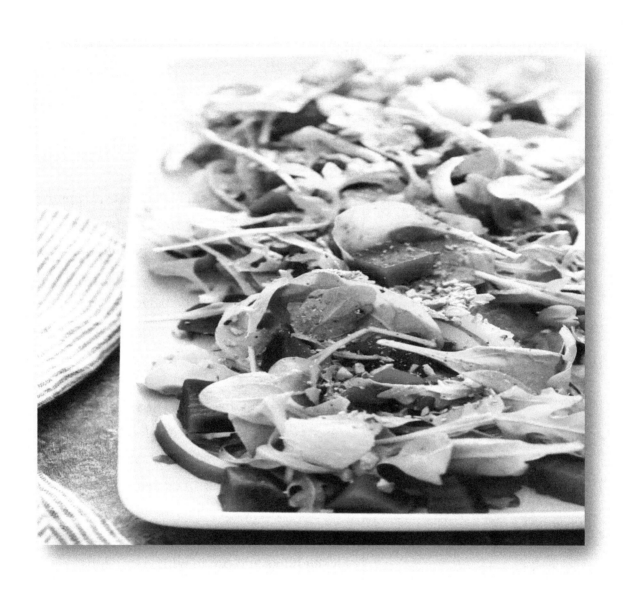

VEGAN CHICKEN

Vegan chicken, one of the best recipes I've ever tried. It's super flavorful, comforting, high in protein, and made with only 9 simple ingredients!

MAKES 8 SERVING/ TOTAL TIME 50 MINUTE

INGREDIENTS

For the vegan chicken:

12 oz firm tofu (340 g)

2 tbsp nutritional yeast

2 tsp garlic powder

2 tsp onion powder

2 tsp chicken seasoning

1 tsp salt

¾ cup vegan chicken stock (180 ml)

1 and ½ cups vital wheat gluten (180 g)

For cooking:

Extra-virgin olive oil or vegan butter

Chicken seasoning to taste

METHOD

STEP 1

Add all the vegan chicken ingredients except the vital wheat gluten to a blender and blend until smooth. Set aside. Transfer to a large bowl and add the vital wheat gluten. Mix until well combined. Make a ball with the dough. It doesn't have to be perfect as it won't change the flavor or texture, it will just make your vegan chicken more beautiful.

STEP 2

Transfer the ball to a cutting board and flatten it out, then cut into 4 pieces. Let the pieces cool down for a few minutes so you don't burn your hands. Unwrap them from the foil and cut each piece lengthways down the middle so that you have 8 pieces.

Sprinkle some chicken seasoning onto the vegan chicken fillets and rub in with your hands.

Heat some extra-virgin olive oil or some vegan butter in a skillet and cook the vegan chicken fillets over medium-high heat until golden brown for both sides. Serve immediately with some lemon wedges, a sauce like vegan mayo,

NUTRITION VALUE

167 Energy, 2.3g fat, 0.4g saturated fat, 1.1g fiber, 22.1g protein, 14.2g carbs.

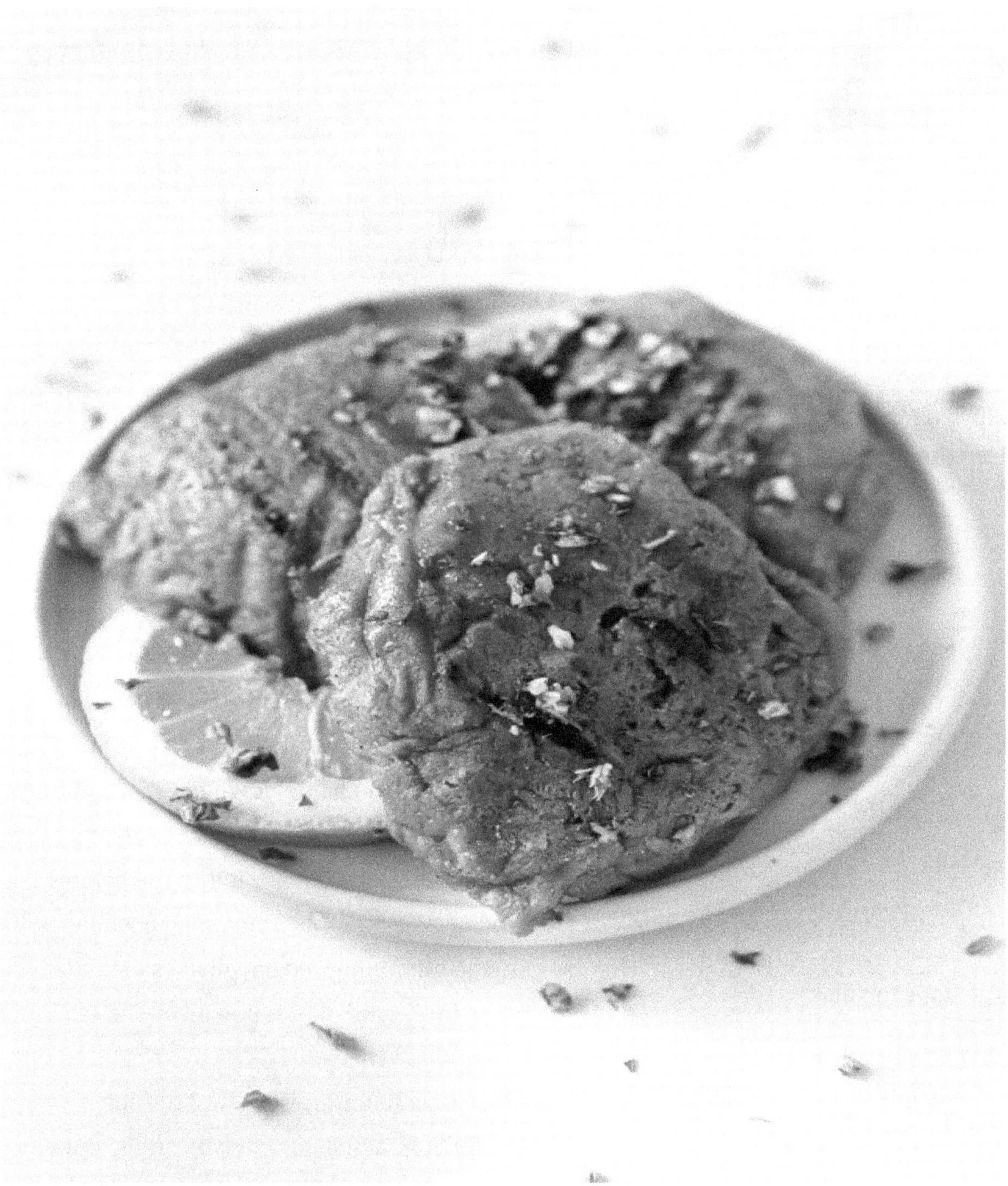

VEGAN ENCHILADAS

Vegan enchiladas, an absolutely delicious and easy Mexican recipe perfect to enjoy for lunch or dinner. Everyone will love them!

MAKES 8 SERVING/ TOTAL TIME 1 HOUR

INGREDIENTS

2 cups butternut squash (400 g), peeled and cubed

2 tbsp extra-virgin olive oil

½ onion, finely chopped

1 15-ounce can black beans (425 g), drained and rinsed

1 4-ounce can diced green chiles (115 g)

1 tsp ground cumin

1 tsp dried oregano

½ tsp salt

¼ tsp ground black pepper

8 large flour tortillas

1 batch homemade red enchilada sauce, or 1 and ¾ cups of store-bought (440 ml)

METHOD

STEP 1

Preheat the oven to 350ºF or 180ºC. Steam or boil the butternut squash for 10 to 15 minutes or until tender. In the meantime, add the oil to a large skillet and cook over medium-high heat until hot. Add the onion and cook until golden brown. Stir to combine and cook for 5 minutes, stirring occasionally. Set aside.

To assemble the vegan enchiladas, spread 6-8 tbsp of red enchilada sauce onto a large baking dish

Lay out a tortilla, and spread 2 tablespoons of sauce over the surface of the tortilla. Add ⅛ of the squash and black bean filling in a line down the center of the tortilla, then sprinkle with some cheese.

Roll up the tortilla and place it into the baking dish, seal side down. Assemble the remaining enchiladas. Then spread the remaining red enchilada sauce evenly over the top of the enchiladas, followed by the remaining vegan shredded cheese.

Bake for 20 to 30 minutes or until the cheese is melted and the tortillas are slightly crispy on the outside.

Serve immediately with a side of cauliflower rice or veggie stir fry.

NUTRITION VALUE	307 Energy, 5.9g fat, 0.8g saturated fat, 13g fiber, 13.5g protein, 52.4g carbs.

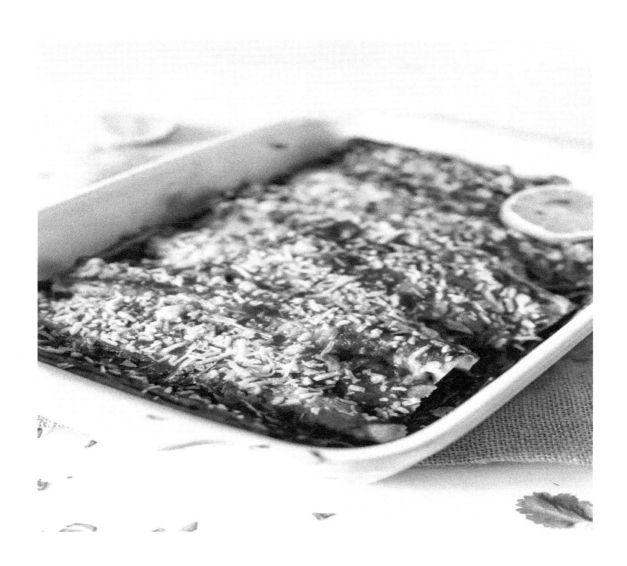

Snacks

VEGAN MASHED SWEET POTATOES

7-ingredient vegan mashed sweet potatoes. They're so tasty, smooth, creamy and ready in about 30 minutes. It's the perfect side dish!

MAKES 4 SERVING/ TOTAL TIME 30 MINUTE

INGREDIENTS

2 pounds sweet potato (900 g)

1/4 cup plant milk of your choice, we used soy milk (65 ml)

2 tbsp maple syrup

2 tbsp nutritional yeast

1 tsp garlic powder

1/2 tsp sea salt

1/8 tsp ground black pepper

Chopped walnuts and dried dill for topping (optional)

METHOD

STEP 1

Peal and dice the sweet potatoes and steam (or boil) them for about 20 to 25 minutes or until they're soft. Add the steamed sweet potatoes to a large mixing bowl with the rest of the ingredients and mash. We used an immersion blender, but feel free to use a potato masher, a fork or even a regular blender.

Top with some chopped walnuts and dried dill (optional) and serve.

NUTRITION VALUE

322 Energy, 1g fat, 0.2g saturated fat, 10.7g fiber, 6.4g protein, 73.8g carbs.

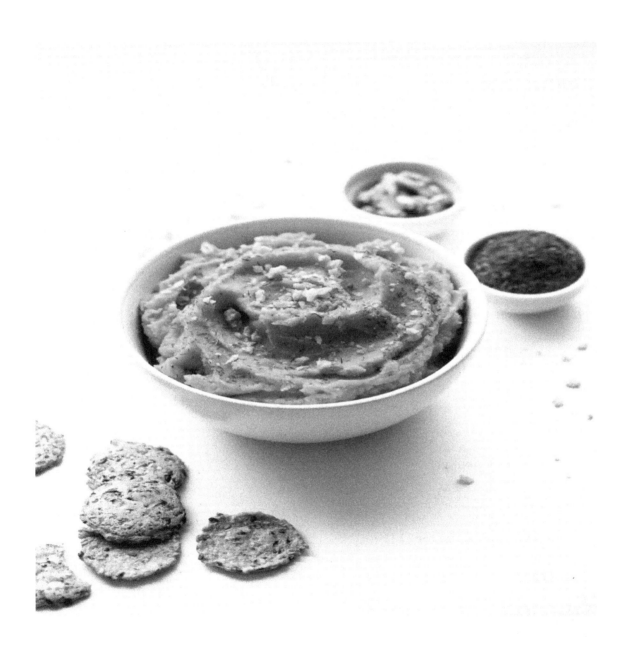

CABBAGE SOUP

Cabbage soup, a tasty and easy way to include more veggies into your diet, It's comforting, super flavorful, and made with extra healthy ingredients!

MAKES 4 SERVING/ TOTAL TIME 40 MINUTE

INGREDIENTS

1 tbsp extra-virgin olive oil

2 cloves of garlic, chopped

1 celery strip, chopped

1/2 onion, chopped

1 carrot, chopped

1/2 red bell pepper, chopped

1 pound cabbage (450 g), chopped

1 tbsp Italian seasoning (optional)

1/2 tsp salt

1/4 tsp ground black pepper

2 bay leaves

4 cups vegetable stock or water (1 l)

1 14-ounce can have crushed tomatoes (400 g)

METHOD

STEP 1

Heat the oil in a large pot and add the garlic, celery, and onion. Cook over medium-high heat for about 5 minutes or until golden brown.

STEP 2

Add all the remaining ingredients and bring to a boil. Then simmer for 30 minutes.
Remove the bay leaves and serve immediately with vegan meat like tempeh, seitan, tofu, vegan bacon, or tempeh bacon, among others. I also add some chopped, fresh parsley on top right before serving.

NUTRITION VALUE

72 Energy, 2.6g fat, 0.4g saturated fat, 3.8g fiber, 2.4g protein, 12g carbs.

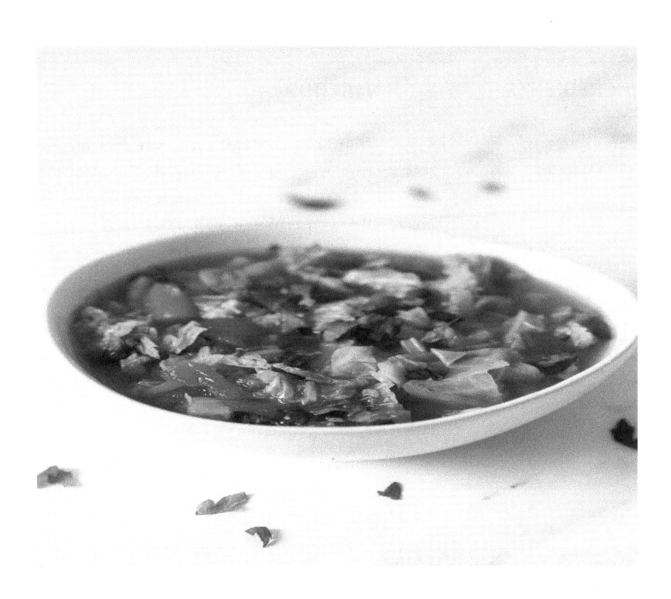

SWEET POTATO HASH

Sweet potato hash, a delicious, healthy, and super easy-to-make side dish that only requires 8 nutritious and affordable ingredients and just 25 minutes!

MAKES 2 SERVING/ TOTAL TIME 25 MINUTE

INGREDIENTS

1–2 tbsp extra-virgin olive oil

1-pound sweet potatoes (450 g), cubed

2 cloves of garlic, chopped

1/2 red onion, chopped

1/2 red bell pepper, chopped

1/2 green bell pepper, chopped

1/2 tsp salt

1/4 tsp ground black pepper

METHOD

STEP 1

Heat the oil in a skillet, add the sweet potato cubes, cover with a lid, and cook over medium heat for about 10 minutes, stirring occasionally. You don't need to peel the sweet potatoes if you don't want to.

Add all the remaining ingredients, stir, uncover, and cook over medium-high heat for about 10 to 15 minutes or until tender and golden brown.

Serve immediately (I added some chopped fresh parsley on top) with some chopped tempeh, seitan, tempeh bacon, or even vegan bacon.

NUTRITION VALUE

142 Energy, 3.5g fat, 0.5g saturated fat, 3.5g fiber, 1.7g protein, 26.9g carbs.

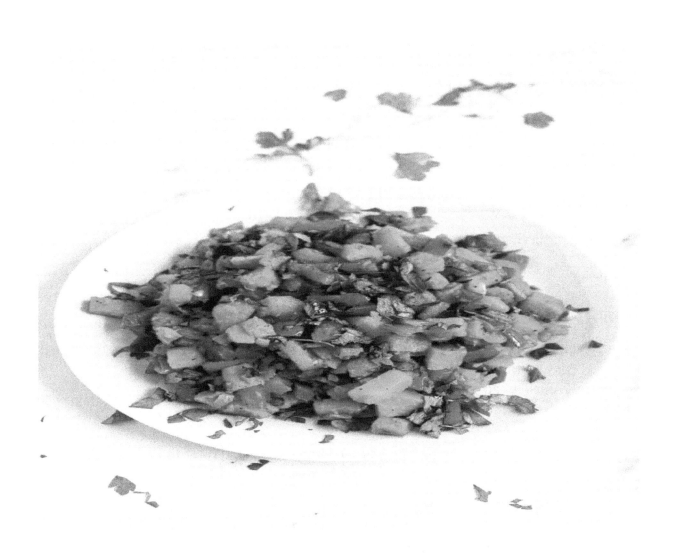

BRUSCHETTA

Bruschetta, a classic Italian appetizer. It's so tasty, simple, made with 8 natural and healthy ingredients, and ready in just 15 minutes.

MAKES 30 SERVING/ TOTAL TIME 15 MINUTE

INGREDIENTS

3 medium tomatoes, diced

1–2 tbsp red onion, finely chopped

1 clove of garlic, minced

2 tbsp fresh basil, chopped

1/4 tsp salt

1/8 tsp ground black pepper

1 tbsp extra-virgin olive oil

1 baguette, French bread or similar Italian bread

METHOD

STEP 1

Combine the tomatoes, onion, garlic, basil, salt, pepper, and oil in a large mixing bowl. Feel free to add more or less oil. Set aside.

STEP 2

Use a bread knife to slice the bread on the diagonal, making 1/2- or 3/4-inch-thick slices (about 1 to 2 cm). Toast the bread. I always use a griddle but feel free to use a grill pan, a skillet, a toaster, the oven, etc. Some people add some oil to the bread before toasting it, but I think that's not necessary.

Place the bread on a platter and top with the tomato mixture.

Serve immediately and toast the bread right before serving.

NUTRITION VALUE	38 Energy, 0.6g fat, 0.1g saturated fat, 0.4g fiber, 1.1g protein, 5.3g carbs.

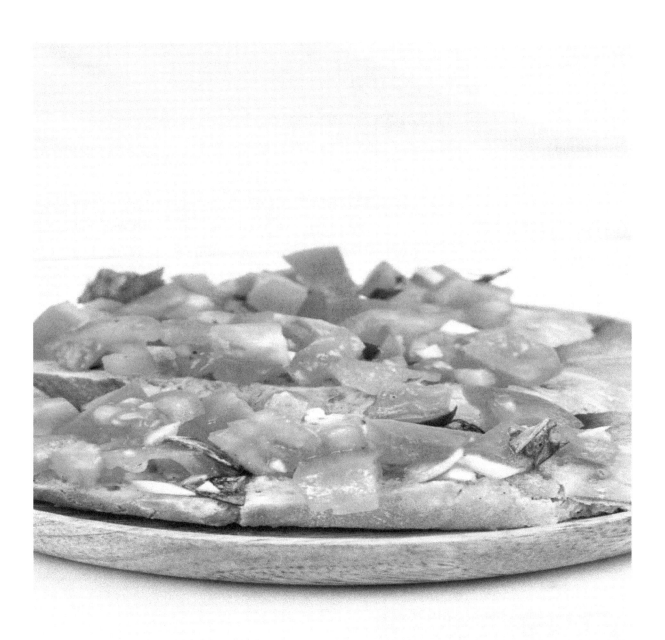

WHITE SANGRIA

White sangria is a sweet and refreshing version of traditional sangria. It's made in 15 minutes with 9 ingredients and it's perfect for the hot summer days!

MAKES 4 SERVING/ TOTAL TIME 15 MINUTE

INGREDIENTS

3 cups white wine (750 ml)

1/2 cup orange juice (125 ml)

2 tbsp Cointreau or brandy (optional)

1 tbsp lemon juice

1/2 cup sugar (90 g), I used brown sugar

2 cinnamon sticks

1 orange, sliced

1 lemon, sliced

1 cup strawberries (150 g), chopped

METHOD

STEP 1

Put the white wine, orange juice, Cointreau, lemon juice, and sugar in a pitcher and mix until well combined. Incorporate the cinnamon sticks and the fruit and stir again.

STEP 2

It's best to let it marinate for at least 30 minutes before serving, but you can serve immediately as well.

Drink it during a dinner with friends and accompany it with baked zucchinis fries, Spanish patatas bravas, pasta salad, or portobello steaks. White sangria goes with plenty of different dishes!

NUTRITION VALUE	146 Energy, 0.2g fat, 1.2g fiber, 0.6g protein, 17.7g carbs.

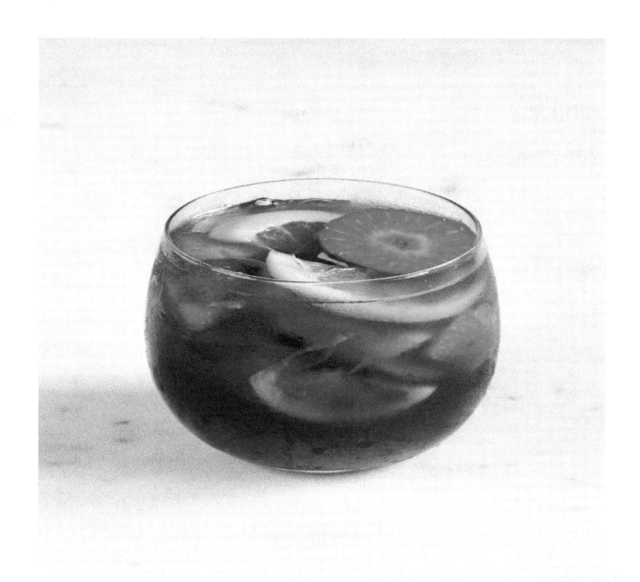

CHICKPEA CREPES

Chickpea crepes are a great vegan and gluten-free alternative to classic crepes and they're so delicious with savory toppings. Only 4 ingredients needed!

MAKES 6 SERVING/ TOTAL TIME 20 MINUTE

INGREDIENTS

1 cup chickpea flour (130 g)

1 and 1/4 cups water (315 ml)

1 tbsp lemon juice

1/2 tsp salt

METHOD

STEP 1

Mix all the ingredients in a mixing bowl until well combined. Feel free to use a blender if you want.

Let the mixture stand in the fridge for 30 minutes.

Heat a non-stick skillet (or a lightly greased skillet) over medium heat.

STEP 2

Pour about ¼ cup (4 tbsp) of the batter onto the pan, twirling the batter around to cover the whole bottom of the pan. I used an 8 inch or 20 cm skillet, so add more or less batter if needed.

Cook for about one minute or until the batter gets darker, loosen the edges with a butter knife and flip the crepe.

Cook for about one minute more until brown the other side of the crepe. Repeat with the remaining batter.

Serve immediately with your favorite toppings

NUTRITION VALUE

79 Energy, 1.3g fat, 0.2g saturated fat, 3.8g fiber, 4.2g protein, 14.2g carbs.

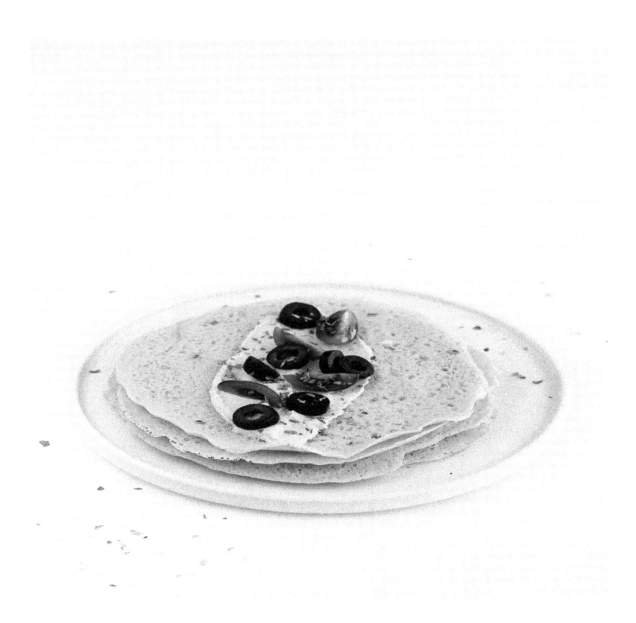

SPANISH GAZPACHO

Gazpacho is a soup made of raw vegetables and served cold. We eat it especially during the hot summers because is so refreshing.

MAKES 6 SERVING/ TOTAL TIME 10 MINUTE

INGREDIENTS

2.2 lbs. very ripe tomatoes (1 kg)

1 cucumber (180 g)

2 Italian green peppers (230 g)

1 clove of garlic (remove the germ to improve your digestion)

2 tbsp apple cider vinegar

1/3 cup extra-virgin olive oil (75 g)

2 tsp sea salt

METHOD

STEP 1

Chop the veggies and place them with the rest of the ingredients in a blender. Blend until smooth.

Chill gazpacho in the fridge for at least 1 or 2 hours, or until it's really cold.

Serve in individual bowls with some raw veggies (I added chopped tomato, green pepper and cucumber), extra-virgin olive oil and black pepper on top (optional).

NUTRITION VALUE	110 Energy, 9.1g fat, 1.3g saturated fat, 2.2g fiber, 1.6g protein, 7.7g carbs.

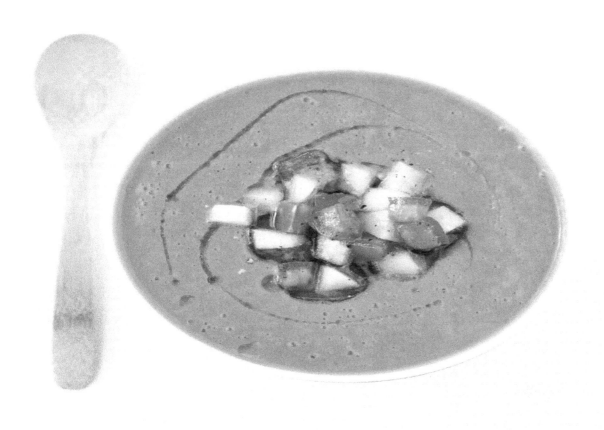

VEGAN BROCCOLI CHEESE SOUP

This vegan broccoli cheese soup is super tasty, simple, low in fat and good for your body. It's the perfect lunch recipe for the fall and winter months.

MAKES 4 SERVING/ TOTAL TIME 35 MINUTE

INGREDIENTS

2 cups potatoes (360 g)

1 cup carrots (135 g)

1/2 cup broccoli florets (250 g)

2 cups vegetable stock (500 ml)

1 cup unsweetened plant milk of your choice (250 ml), we used soy milk

1/2 cup nutritional yeast (35 g)

1 tbsp lemon juice

1 tsp sea salt

1/2 tsp garlic powder

1/2 tsp onion powder

1/8 tsp ground black pepper

METHOD

STEP 1

Peel and chop the potatoes and carrots and steam (or boil) them for 20 minutes or until soft.

In the meanwhile, steam (or boil) the broccoli florets for 5 to 10 minutes or until soft.

When the veggies are cooked, add them to a blender with the rest of the ingredients and blend until smooth. Cook the soup in a large pot over medium-high heat for 5 minutes.

Serve and top with your favorite ingredients (we added some baked croutons and chopped fresh parsley).

NUTRITION VALUE

184 Energy, 2.3g fat, 0.3g saturated fat, 8.3g fiber, 13.1g protein, 31.4g carbs.

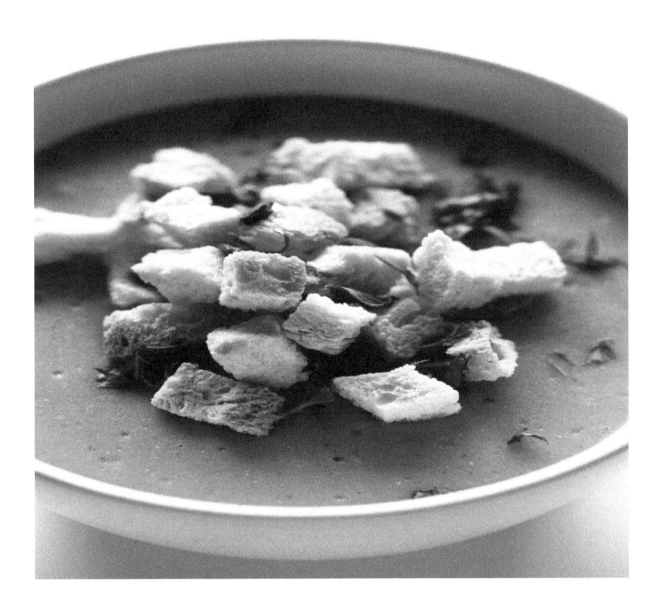

VEGAN CHOCOLATE ORANGE TRUFFLES

These vegan chocolate orange truffles are ready in 15 minutes or even less and are a super healthy treat or snack.

MAKES 16 SERVING/ TOTAL TIME 15 MINUTE

INGREDIENTS

1 cup Medjool dates, pitted (200 g)

1/2 cup almond meal (50 g)

2 tbsp unsweetened cocoa powder + extra cocoa powder for rolling the balls in

2 tbsp orange juice

Zest of 1 orange

METHOD

STEP 1

Place all the ingredients in a food processor or a powerful blender and blend until well combined. Make balls with your hands. We made 16 truffles. Finally, roll the truffles in some cocoa powder. This step is optional.

You can store them in a sealed container in the fridge for about 2 weeks or freeze them for months.

NUTRITION VALUE

58 Energy, 1.9g fat, 0.2g saturated fat, 1.5g fiber, 1.2g protein, 10.6g carbs.

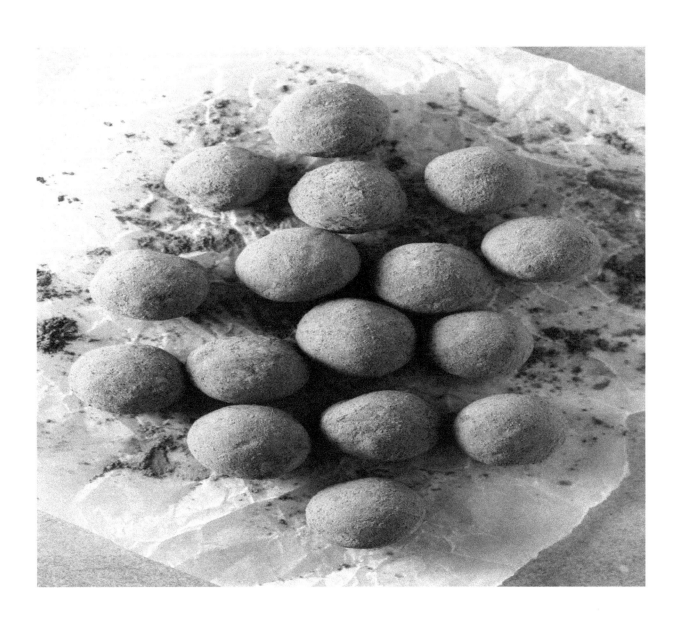

VEGAN SLOPPY JOES

Vegan Sloppy Joes, delicious and easy to make. They're ready in just 30 minutes and require simple ingredients, and they're packed with lots of protein!

MAKES 6 SERVING/ TOTAL TIME 30 MINUTE

INGREDIENTS

1–2 tbsp extra-virgin olive oil

1/8 tsp cayenne powder (optional)

2 cloves of garlic, chopped

1/4 onion, chopped

1/2 red bell pepper, chopped

1/2 green bell pepper, chopped

15 oz canned or cooked lentils (400 g)

1 1/2 cup tomato sauce (250 g)

2 tbsp soy sauce or tamari

2 tbsp tomato paste

1 tbsp brown sugar

2 tsp garlic powder

2 tsp onion powder

1 tsp sweet paprika

METHOD

STEP 1

Heat the oil in a pan and add the veggies and the cayenne powder. Cook over medium-high heat until golden brown, stirring occasionally. Add more oil or a little bit of water if needed.

STEP 2

Add all the remaining ingredients, stir, and cook for about 10 minutes or until the sauce thickens.

Serve the filling over the buns and add your favorite veggies (I added some red cabbage, carrot, fresh chili peppers, and avocado slices).

Keep the leftover filling in an airtight container in the fridge for 3-5 days or in the freezer for up to 3 months.

NUTRITION VALUE	1190 KJ Energy, 8.7g fat, 1.9g saturated fat, 13.6g fiber, 11.3g protein, 32.2g carbs.

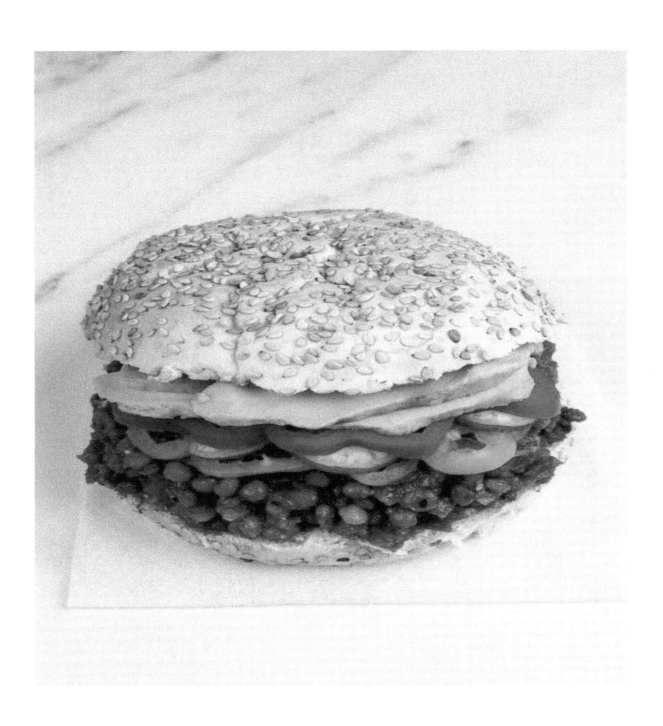

Desserts

VEGAN TORRIJAS

Vegan Torrijas. Torrijas is a typical Spanish dessert of Lent and Holy Week, and they are very similar to French toast. You're going to love it!

MAKES 14 SERVING/ TOTAL TIME 30 MINUTE

INGREDIENTS

2 cups almond milk (500 milliliters)

1/2 cinnamon stick

Lemon zest

8 tablespoons brown sugar + extra sugar to sprinkle on top

5.6 oz or 160 grams of bread

4 tablespoons of chickpea flour

4 tablespoons water

Extra-virgin olive oil

METHOD

STEP 1

Cut the bread into slices 1/2 or 3/4 inches (one or two centimeters) thick.

In a saucepan, heat the milk with cinnamon and lemon zest. When they are hot, add 8 tablespoons of brown sugar, cook for 3 or 4 minutes and remove from heat. Put the bread slices on a rectangular dish (we used a glass roaster) and pour the mixture over the bread. Let set at least 5 minutes on each side to absorb the milk, although you have to be careful that they are not too soft because they could break. Depending on the type of bread that you're using, you will have to leave more or less time.

STEP 2

On a plate or bowl, mix 4 tablespoons of chickpea flour with 4 tablespoons of water. Soak the torrijas in the mixture and fry in a pan with hot oil until golden brown on both sides.

Sprinkle brown sugar on top and let cool the torrijas.

NUTRITION VALUE

283 Energy, 11.5g fat, 1.6g saturated fat, 2.9g fiber, 2.3g protein, 43.2g carbs.

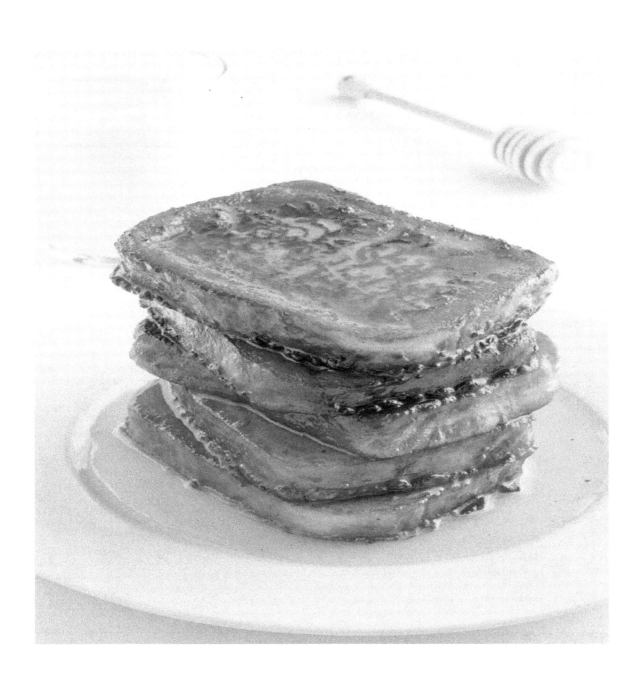

VEGAN GLUTEN FREE SPANISH CHOCOLATE POLVORONES

These vegan, gluten-free Spanish chocolate polvorones are a healthy alternative to traditional polvorones (made with lard, sugar, and white flour.)

MAKES 22 SERVING/ TOTAL TIME 50 MINUTE

INGREDIENTS

¾ cup raw almonds (120 g)

1 ¾ cup buckwheat flour (240 g)

¾ cup oat flour (90 g)

4 tbsp unsweetened cocoa powder or raw cacao

1 cup extra-virgin olive oil (220 g)

½ cup coconut sugar (130 g)

½ cup maple syrup (160 g)

Sesame seeds

METHOD

STEP 1

Preheat the oven to 355ºF or 180ºC.

Blend the almonds in a food processor.

Add the rest of the ingredients (except the sesame seeds) and blend until well combined

Shape the polvorones with your hands and add some sesame seeds on top.

Place them onto a baking sheet (I lined it with parchment paper) and bake for 30 minutes or until golden brown.

NUTRITION VALUE

1190 KJ Energy, 8.7g fat, 1.9g saturated fat, 13.6g fiber, 11.3g protein, 32.2g carbs.

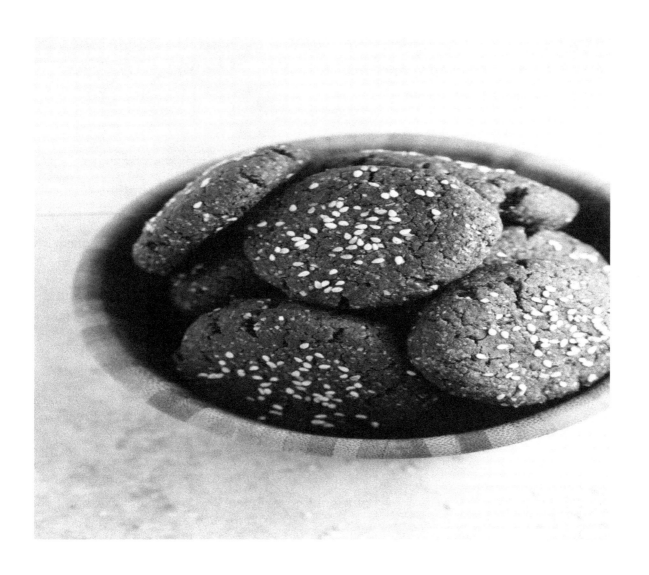

VEGAN GLUTEN FREE CHOCOLATE CAKE (10 MINUTES)

Vegan gluten-free chocolate cake, made with 6 ingredients in just than 10 minutes! It's also so delicious, super healthy and low in fat. You can eat it for breakfast, as a dessert or a snack.

MAKES 2 SERVING/ TOTAL TIME 10 MINUTE

INGREDIENTS

For the cake:

- 1/2 banana
- 6 tbsp full-fat coconut milk
- 4 tbsp cane, coconut or brown sugar
- 4 tbsp flour, we used buckwheat flour
- 2 tbsp unsweetened cocoa powder
- 1/2 tsp baking soda

For the peanut butter frosting (optional):

- 3 tbsp full-fat coconut milk
- 2 tbsp peanut butter

METHOD

STEP 1

Add the half banana to a mixing bowl and mash it with a fork.

Then add the rest of the ingredients and stir until well mixed. You can also blend all the ingredients in a blender to get a smoother texture, but it's not necessary.

Place the bowl in a side of the microwave, not in the center and cook for 4 minutes.

STEP 2

Remove from the microwave and let the cake cool down at room temperature. Feel free to enjoy it hot if you want.

To make the peanut butter frosting, just mix the ingredients in a bowl until well combined and add it on top of the cake and some chopped peanuts as well (optional). We didn't add all the frosting to the cake for the pictures, but we ate it all with the cake.

NUTRITION VALUE

130 KJ Energy, 6g fat, 5.1g saturated fat, 2.5g fiber, 2.2g protein, 20.2g carbs.

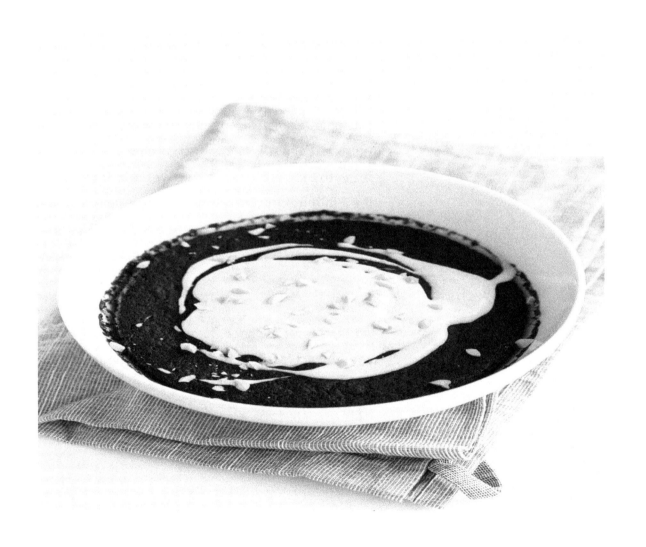

CARAMBOLAS IN GREEN TEA AND GINGER SYRUP

Green tea is well known for its health benefits. It tastes delicious too in this stylish and refreshing dessert.

MAKES 6 SERVING/ TOTAL TIME 27 MINUTE

INGREDIENTS

500ml (2 cups) water

115g (1/2 cup) caster sugar

5cm piece fresh ginger, peeled, thinly sliced

30g (1/4 cup) green tea leaves

3 large (about 450g) carambolas (star fruit), cut crossways into 1cm-thick slices

6 scoops lemon sorbet (Weis brand)

METHOD
STEP 1
Place the water, sugar and ginger in a medium saucepan. Cook over low heat, stirring, for 2 minutes or until the sugar dissolves. Increase heat to high and bring to the boil. Simmer, uncovered, without stirring, for 5 minutes or until syrup thickens slightly. Remove from heat and stir in the tea. Set aside for 5 minutes to infuse. Strain through a fine sieve into a large heatproof bowl.

STEP 2
Add the carambolas to the ginger syrup and stir until combined. Place in the fridge for 10 minutes to develop the flavors.

STEP 3
Divide the carambolas among shallow serving bowls and drizzle with some of the syrup. Top with a scoop of sorbet and serve immediately.

NUTRITION VALUE

545 KJ Energy, 8.7g fat,
1g protein, 29g carbs.

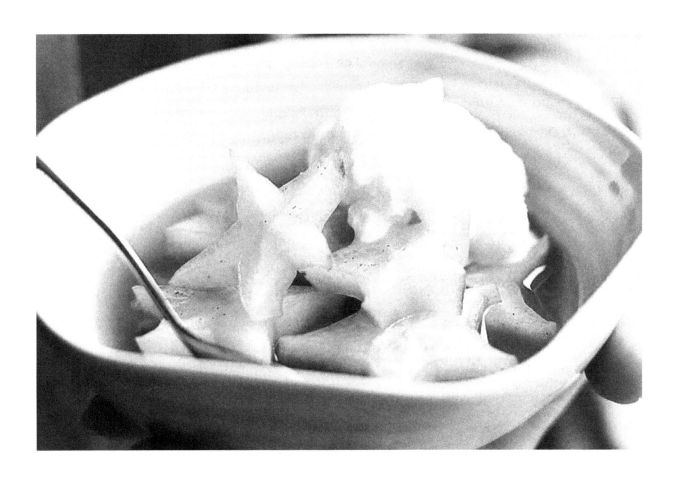

VEGAN PEPPERMINT SLICE

A delightful **vegan** sweet treat that is lower in calories. This recipe does take a little time, but the reward is worth it.

MAKES 24 SERVING/ TOTAL TIME 13 HOUR 30 MINUTE

INGREDIENTS

1 tablespoon white quinoa

2 1/2 tablespoons coconut oil

90g (1 cup) rolled oats

2 tablespoons raw cacao powder

100g fresh dates, pitted, chopped

PEPPERMINT FILLING

290g (2 cups) cashews

140ml can coconut milk

100g (1/4 cup) rice malt syrup

20g (1/4 cup) desiccated coconut

2 tablespoons coconut oil

2 teaspoons peppermint extract

CHOCOLATE TOPPING

50g (1/2 cup) raw cacao powder, sifted

185g (1/2 cup) rice malt syrup

110g (1/2 cup) coconut oil

METHOD

STEP 1

Preheat oven to 180C/160C fan forced. Line a baking tray with baking paper. Grease the base and sides of a 16 x 26cm (base measurement) slice pan and line with baking paper. Toss quinoa and 1 tsp melted coconut oil together in a bowl. Spread the oats and quinoa mixture over prepared tray. Bake, stirring halfway, for 8-10 minutes or until golden. Cool completely.

STEP 2

Process cashews in the food processor until smooth. Add 2 tbs thick coconut milk from the top of the can. Add syrup, desiccated coconut, coconut oil and extract. Process well, scraping the sides, until well combined. Spread over oat base and use a spatula to smooth the surface. Place in the fridge for 2 hours or until firm. For the chocolate topping, place ingredients in a heatproof bowl set over a saucepan of simmering .Cook, stirring constantly, for 4 minutes , Place in the fridge for 6 hours or overnight to set. Cut slice into 24 squares.

NUTRITION VALUE

928 KJ Energy, 15.4g fat, 9.3g saturated fat, 2.5g fiber, 8g protein, 21.3g carbs.

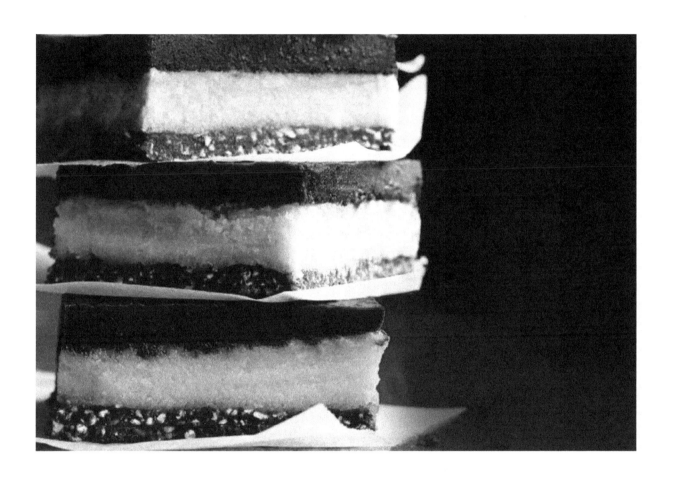

VEGAN ICE CREAM

Vegan ice cream, sweet and delicious. With a smooth texture, it's made with 10 easy-to-find ingredients. It is completely dairy-free and so good!

MAKES 10 SERVING/ TOTAL TIME 50 MINUTE

INGREDIENTS

1 cup raw and unsalted cashews (150 g)

1 vanilla bean, optional

1 cup water (250 ml)

1 cup sugar (200 g), I used refined white sugar

1/4 cup water (64 ml)

1/2 cup cocoa butter (60 g)

1/4 cup coconut oil (65 ml)

1/2 tsp salt

1 cup coconut milk (250 ml)

2 tsp vanilla extract

METHOD

STEP 1

Soak the cashews overnight at room temperature. You could also soak them in hot water for at least 1 hour, although the ice cream's texture will be better if you do it overnight. Cut the vanilla bean in half lengthwise and scrape it to take off the seeds. Reserve.

STEP 2

Drain and rinse the cashews and add them into a blender with 1 cup of water (250 ml). Blend until well combined. Cook the sugar and water in a saucepan over medium heat for 1 or 2 minutes, stirring occasionally. Incorporate the coconut oil, cocoa butter, and salt, stir and cook over medium heat until well mixed. Keep stirring. Mix the cashews and water in a bowl with the coconut milk.

STEP 3

Incorporate the mixture of sugar, water, coconut oil, cocoa butter, and salt, and also the vanilla extract and the vanilla seeds. Whisk or blend until well combined. Keep the bowl in the freezer for 1 hour. Get creative and enjoy it with your favorite toppings!

NUTRITION VALUE	310 KJ Energy, 5.6g fat, 13.5g saturated fat, 0.5g fiber, 2.9g protein, 25.4g carbs.

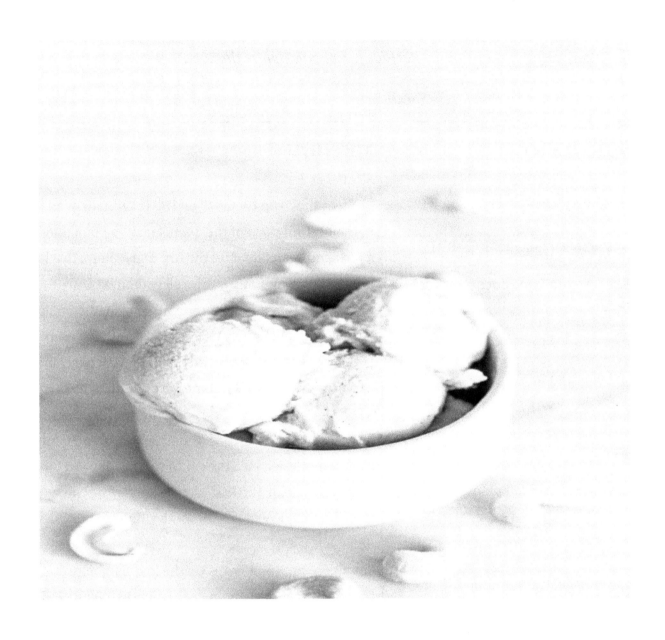

SIMPLE VEGAN BANANA BREAD

This is the best vegan banana bread ever! Sweet, moist in the inside, crispy on the outside, and full of flavor. Perfect for breakfast or dessert.

MAKES 12 SERVING/ TOTAL TIME 70 MINUTE

INGREDIENTS

1 and 1/2 cups mashed very ripe bananas (about 3 large bananas)

2 cups whole wheat flour (240 g)

3/4 cup brown, cane or coconut sugar (135 g)

1 tsp ground cinnamon

1 tsp baking soda

1/4 tsp salt

1 flax egg

1/2 cup unsweetened plant milk of your choice (125 ml), I used soy milk

1/3 cup coconut oil (85 ml), melted

1 tsp vanilla extract, optional

METHOD

STEP 1

Preheat the oven to 350°F or 180ºC with an oven rack in the bottom third of the oven. Mash the bananas with a fork and set aside. Add the dry ingredients to a large mixing bowl and mix until well combined.

Add all the remaining ingredients (mashed bananas, flax egg, oil and vanilla extract). Stir until well mixed.

Line a 9×5-inch (23×13 cm) loaf pan with parchment paper or grease it with some coconut oil.

STEP 2

Add the batter to the pan and bake for 60 to 70 minutes Stick a toothpick into the center of the loaf and if it comes out clean, the loaf is done. Cover the top with foil if the banana bread gets browned, but the middle isn't done yet.

Let it cool for 15 minutes on the loaf pan before transferring it to a cooling rack and then let it cool completely.

NUTRITION VALUE

204 KJ Energy, 8g fat, 7g saturated fat, 3.7g fiber, 3.7g protein, 31.7g carbs.

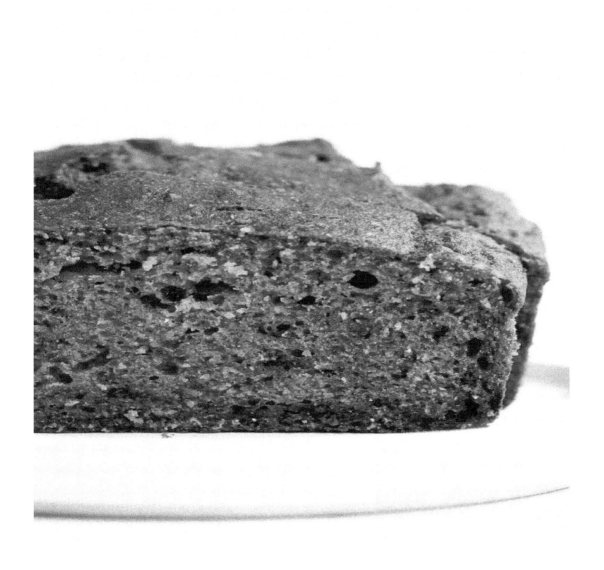

VEGAN GRILLED PINEAPPLE SUNDAES

If you're looking for a delicious and easy to make dessert, these vegan grilled pineapple sundaes are for you. Only 4 ingredients required!

MAKES 4 SERVING/ TOTAL TIME 15 MINUTE

INGREDIENTS

4 pineapple slices

Vegan vanilla ice cream

Homemade chocolate syrup

Coconut chips (optional)

METHOD

STEP 1

I prefer to use fresh pineapple to make this recipe, but canned is also okay. Fresh pineapple slices are bigger and take longer to cook than the canned ones. If you use fresh pineapple, you may want to remove the core if it's really hard (I didn't).

Grill the pineapple slices until charred (no oil needed). Top each pineapple slice with vegan vanilla ice cream and drizzle with some homemade chocolate syrup. Top with coconut chips and serve immediately.

NUTRITION VALUE

135 Energy, 5.4g fat, 2.9g saturated fat, 0.9g fiber, 1.7g protein, 21.5g carbs.

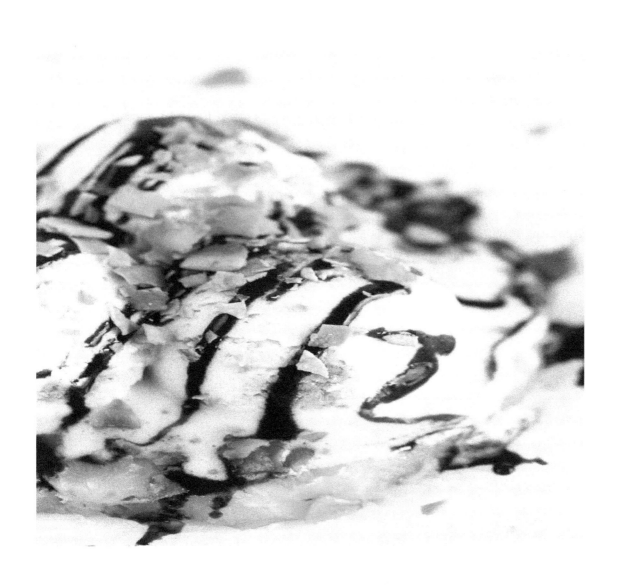

VEGAN CASHEW FROSTING

This delicious vegan cashew frosting is super healthy and so simple and easy to make. You can use it to make cakes, cupcakes or any desserts you want.

MAKES 12 SERVING/ TOTAL TIME 15 MINUTE

INGREDIENTS

1 and 1/3 cups unsalted, raw cashews (200 g)

1/2 cup almond milk (125 ml)

2 tbsp agave syrup

1/4 tsp cinnamon powder

1/2 vanilla bean, scraped (optional)

METHOD

STEP 1

Soak the cashews for at least 4 hours, better overnight.

Drain and wash the cashews and place them in a blender with the rest of the ingredients.

Blend until smooth. Add more milk if needed.

Store it in a sealed container in the fridge for up to 4 days.

NUTRITION VALUE

102 Energy, 7.4g fat, 1.3g saturated fat, 0.7g fiber, 3.1g protein, 6.9g carbs.

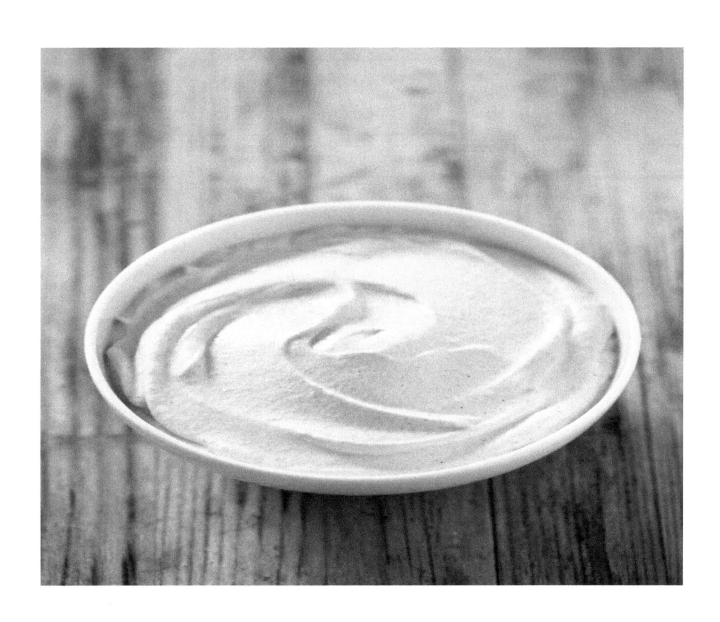

3-INGREDIENT RAW CACAO BITES

If you need to eat something sweet, you should try these 3-ingredient raw cacao bites, they taste so good and you only need 3 ingredients to make them.

MAKES 14 SERVING/ TOTAL TIME 5 MINUTE

INGREDIENTS

1 cup walnuts (115 g)

1 cup Medjool dates (200 g)

2 tbsp raw cacao

METHOD

STEP 1

Place the walnuts in a food processor or a powerful blender (food processors work better) and blend until they have a crumbly texture.

STEP 2

Add the dates and the cacao and blend again.

Make balls with your hands and they're ready to serve.

You can store the bites in a sealed container at room temperature, although I prefer to keep them in the fridge, especially in summer.

NUTRITION VALUE

95 Energy, 5.5g fat, 0.6g saturated fat, 1.8g fiber, 1.7g protein, 12.3g carbs.

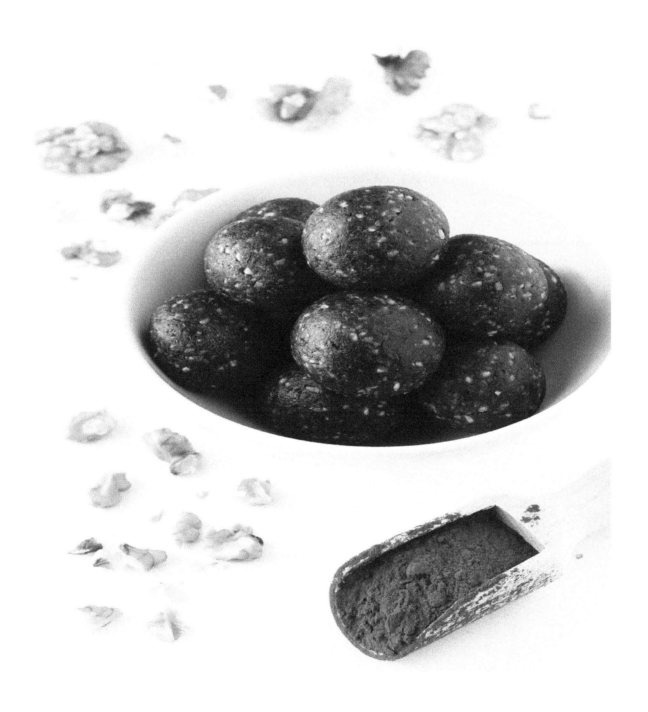

CPSIA information can be obtained
at www.ICGtesting.com
Printed in the USA
LVHW060332110521
687014LV00015B/1379